ROMANCING THE SPERM

ROMANCING THE SPERM

ROMANCING THE SPERM

Shifting Biopolitics and the Making of Modern Families

DIANE TOBER

RUTGERS UNIVERSITY PRESS

New Brunswick, Camden, and Newark, New Jersey, and London

Library of Congress Cataloging-in-Publication Data

Names: Tober, Diane, author.
Title: Romancing the sperm : shifting biopolitics and the making of modern
    families / Diane Tober.
Description: New Brunswick : Rutgers University Press, [2018] | Includes
    bibliographical references and index.
Identifiers: LCCN 2018004643| ISBN 9780813590790 (cloth) |
    ISBN 9780813590783 (pbk.)
Subjects: LCSH: Artificial insemination—Social aspects. | Human reproductive
    technology—Social aspects. | Single mothers. | Families.
Classification: LCC HQ761 .T63 2018 | DDC 618.1/78—dc23
LC record available at https://lccn.loc.gov/2018004643

A British Cataloging-in-Publication record for this book is available from
the British Library.

Copyright © 2019 by Diane Tober
All rights reserved

No part of this book may be reproduced or utilized in any form or by any means,
electronic or mechanical, or by any information storage and retrieval system, without
written permission from the publisher. Please contact Rutgers University Press,
106 Somerset Street, New Brunswick, NJ 08901. The only exception to this prohibition
is "fair use" as defined by U.S. copyright law.

⊖ The paper used in this publication meets the requirements of the American National
Standard for Information Sciences—Permanence of Paper for Printed Library
Materials, ANSI Z39.48-1992.

www.rutgersuniversitypress.org

Manufactured in the United States of America

For my parents, who stand by me every step of the way, and for my sons, who make life more meaningful

CONTENTS

PREFACE

This book explores how single women and lesbian couples created their families, on their own terms, in the 1990s. Some women purchased sperm from sperm banks; some approached men they knew to be sperm donors. Some women were just starting the process of trying to conceive, some were successful and were either pregnant or raising children, and others were unsuccessful, following years of failed infertility treatments. This project is an attempt to lend a sensitive ear and a compelling voice to what women go through when attempting to conceive a child on their own or with a female partner—especially in light of the social, medical, legal, and political environments that marginalized families created outside heterosexual nuclear family structures, which are commonly viewed as the norm.

Language around sex, sexuality, and gender has changed dramatically since I first started this work. At the time, terms like *cisgender woman* or *trans woman* or *masculine identified* did not exist. All participants in my study were either in a couple or single, considered themselves women, and were lesbian, bisexual, or heterosexual. Some who were lesbian or bisexual identified would also identify as "dyke," "butch," "femme," and so on. I try to be as specific as possible in respect to how people identify themselves throughout my work. Since I did not have trans people in my initial research sample, I am using the terms that were appropriate at that time. I do not intend to marginalize transgender identities or reproductive experiences, but these were not part of my study; however, they are worthy of further research. As an anthropologist, it is important to stay as close as possible to people's own categories and self-identifications. Where appropriate, I do include discussions of trans identities and experiences.

Participants in this research repeatedly asked me two questions: Are you lesbian? I am not. Do you have kids? The answer to the second question is more complicated, and it changed throughout the course of my research. I assume the people I spoke to over the course of this research wanted to know my position regarding both them and the research I was conducting. While this research started off as an interesting anthropological project that would fulfill the requirements for my doctoral degree in the University of California, Berkeley/University of California, San Francisco, medical anthropology program, over the course of many years, it turned deeply personal.

I came to this project through my work as a research assistant on a National Institutes of Health–funded project exploring gender differences in response to infertility, led by medical anthropologist Gay Becker and reproductive endocrinologist Robert Nachtigall. For this project I ventured into people's homes, and into their private lives, in order to uncover the struggles heterosexual couples face when dealing with infertility. Many of the stories I heard were tragic: there were numerous accounts of miscarriages, stillbirths, ectopic pregnancies, botched surgeries, and couples' life savings spent on infertility treatment. It seemed the lengths people would go to in order to have a biological child were extreme. Yet the few who were successful in conceiving and delivering a healthy baby considered the emotional, physical, and financial sacrifices to be worth it.

Throughout my research, I attended many infertility support groups through Resolve, a national organization that provides support and resources for people with infertility. As a single woman myself at the time, I soon realized that most of the symposiums and groups targeted heterosexual married couples. In 1991, at a Resolve conference at Mills College, I overheard a lesbian couple complain that there was no relevant information regarding the issues they were facing in their quest to conceive a child. I then realized that a study of women attempting to conceive without male partners needed to be done.

At the same time, single women and lesbian couples were calling to volunteer to be research subjects for the University of California, San Francisco, study, but they were turned away because they did not fit the parameters of the study, which was exploring the impact infertility has on married couples and how women and men respond differently. I told Gay of my interest in learning more about women's experiences in having a child without a male partner and asked her if she could refer unmarried women who wanted to participate in the research project to me. As early as 1992, I began interviewing women who called to volunteer for the larger study.

From a research perspective, I was interested in two main questions. First, how do sexual orientation, relationship status, and fertility or infertility affect women's identity? This in some ways mirrors the gender differences question in the larger National Institutes of Health–funded study, but without comparative difference from men. The second question was, How do women choose a sperm donor when they are not trying to match a male partner? I figured that women may have different criteria when not trying to match a male partner, and how women chose donors could provide deeper insight into how cultural perceptions of genetic inheritance affect individual reproductive practice. Here, I was thinking in terms of the linkages between culture and biology, and how individual and cultural interpretations of attractiveness, intelligence, creativity, race, health, and other characteristics come to the fore when choosing a donor. I perceived donor choice as a reflection of the kind of children women wanted to bring into their lives.

As I was conducting this research, I found the political and social tensions surrounding single and same-sex family creation to be quite intense. I first became aware of this when several funding agencies critiqued my research proposal for not studying heterosexual couples. They seemed to be missing the point of my research; or maybe they considered this topic too controversial. At the same time, then–California governor Pete Wilson was attempting to pass legislation that would prohibit single men and women and same-sex couples from adopting children. I wondered how such legislation could ultimately affect access to donor insemination and medical treatment for infertility for unmarried women.

When I first started this research, I was also reading Adrienne Rich's *Of Woman Born* (1986) for a seminar on the anthropology of mothering taught by Nancy Scheper-Hughes. This also led me to think about how the family is constructed within American society, and how the notion of the ideal family unit is inextricably bound with compulsory heterosexuality and marriage. As Rich argues, "compulsory heterosexuality" is not "natural" but rather an institution imposed by cultures, societies, and systems that disempower women and keep them subordinate to men (1980).

Yet, as evidenced by the documentation of what was then called "alternative families" in the media (e.g., co-parenting arrangements between lesbian and gay couples, families with same-sex parents, and single mothers by choice), people were challenging the nuclear family model. Reproductive technologies played an integral role in opening up alternative means for the creation of families beyond the institution of heterosexual marriage.

In the fall of 1991, my academic, theoretical interests became personal. I interviewed a woman in Berkeley for the University of California, San Francisco, study. She was thirty-five, and she and her husband had been trying to conceive, unsuccessfully, for five years. During the interview, she turned the tables and started asking me questions: "How old are you?" "Twenty-nine," I responded. "I'll be thirty in two weeks." "When did you have your last pelvic exam?" she asked. When I told her it had been almost three years, as I am one of those people who has always put off going to the doctor, she urged me to schedule an appointment immediately. "Diane," she said, "don't be like me. When I was your age I figured I had plenty of time to have a child. I eat right. I exercise. I'm healthy. I never imagined I would be thirty-five and not able to get pregnant."

I took her words to heart and called the Berkeley Student Health Center to schedule an appointment as soon as I got home from our interview. My appointment fell one day before my thirtieth birthday, in the middle of November 1991. The nurse practitioner determined my uterus seemed malformed and then called in the gynecologist to examine me. They asked me if I was pregnant— I was not—and then determined that I should have an ultrasound to make sure everything was normal.

The following day, I returned to the student health center to get the ultrasound results, which revealed I had two large cysts, one on each ovary. The physician gave me a list of physicians who could perform the surgery to remove the cysts. Because of my research on the infertility project, I had also become familiar with the names and reputations of many specialists in reproductive surgery, many of whom the gynecologist had not mentioned. One doctor, Simon Henderson, kept coming up as an extremely competent and caring surgeon. In fact, the woman I interviewed—who was responsible for encouraging me to go in for my annual exam—had used him. Because of his excellent reputation both in the medical community and among women who had been his patients, I decided he was the right choice.

The physician at the health center was incensed that the surgeon I chose was not a woman. She proceeded to explain to me that women physicians needed the support of women patients, and any gynecologist could do the type of surgery I needed. I explained that while I was certainly sympathetic to the issues facing women in medicine, I could not potentially compromise my future fertility in order to meet her definition of a feminist statement. I found it odd that she was attempting to restrict my decisions concerning my own body. Yet I was torn between my support for women physicians and my knowledge of an excellent microsurgeon who happened to be male. My body had become the site of an external and internal political struggle. As an anthropologist, I interpreted this incident as another example of how women's bodies can become controlled and managed through the medical establishment; yet the educated consumer (with decent medical insurance) can negotiate and assume control over the course of her own treatment.

Within a matter of weeks—through tear-streaked excursions to collect blood samples to test for ovarian cancer, panic attacks, further exams, and sleepless nights—I was scheduled for surgery.

The day after Thanksgiving 1991, I traveled to Children's Hospital in San Francisco with my family. After a morning of intravenous glucose solution, I was prepared for surgery. The anesthesiologist inserted a new concoction into the IV in my hand, and I drifted off into an anesthetized haze, hearing myself discussing the medicalization of women's bodies, the indignity of maintaining brain-dead pregnant women on life support for the sake of the fetus (a paper I had been working on at the time), and similar topics. The surgeon and his staff must have been relieved to have finally silenced this critic and subject of modern medicine so they could perform the required surgery on her docile body.

Awakening, I found out that one ovary had been removed and the other had been completely reconstructed. "One cyst was the size of a small pineapple and the other was the size of a grapefruit," Dr. Henderson told me. *Why are these fruit metaphors being used in reference to my reproductive organs?* I wondered. "The left ovary had no normal ovarian tissue left. The right one was shelled out by the cyst, but we were able to piece it back together." Visions of a shattered Humpty Dumpty egg surrounded by a team of puzzled surgeons passed through my mind. "You are very lucky. Most other surgeons would have just removed both ovaries." *WHAT???* I reached for my side, as if I would be able to make sure that my ovary was still there.

Dr. Henderson seemed very proud of his work. Still hazy from the anesthesia, I was trying to make sense of what he was telling me. Would my ovary work? Would I still be able to have children? These questions could only be answered with time, but this one small portion of my body—that I had never given much consideration other than during the occasional ovulation cramp—suddenly became immense.

During my physical recovery, I became obsessed with my future fertility. After the surgery, I occasionally experienced hot flashes. Each time this happened, I was convinced I was going through premature menopause. I was in a constant panic that my remaining ovary would fail me. I envisioned estrogen replacement therapy, osteoporosis, premature gray hair, and children from another woman's eggs as my future. I told my parents that if I did not have children by the time I was thirty-five—the magic number among most of my research participants—I would use donor insemination to get pregnant and have a child on my own. They seemed to understand, but I felt they would have preferred me to be married before having kids.

My emotional recovery was more prolonged than that of my physical body. After my surgery, I was still conducting interviews for the larger infertility study. All of the sudden, my position as an anthropologist transformed. I shifted from being a distanced observer and gatherer of other people's stories to being able to feel the story of every single person who shared her experience with me. Every interview I did was an agonizing experience. On several occasions, especially when women would discuss their personal tragedies and feelings of loss and failure, my eyes would begin to water and I would choke up, struggling to continue. Many times, upon leaving their houses, I would sit in my car and cry, fearing their stories would someday be my own.

I was on a new mission: to find someone with whom I could have children. Although donor insemination was certainly an option I could have pursued, at this point in my life it seemed too radical a choice for me personally. I could not bring myself to defy the social conventions in which I had been raised. I worried about how my parents would react. How could I justify choosing to become a single mother while I was a financially struggling graduate student? Yet waiting until I finished my PhD seemed too risky a prospect as far as my fertility was concerned. Because of my exposure to infertility through the research, and my witnessing the trauma so many women faced, having children became my primary concern.

I broke off a two-year, headed-nowhere relationship. I quickly met someone else, conceived, married hastily, gave birth to my first child in 1994, and twenty-one months later, in 1995, my second son was born. In the span of four years, aside from when I was visibly pregnant, I was still interviewing people for the gender differences project and my own research. I also went through my own close brush with infertility and, by the end of my graduate studies, a divorce. By 1997, I was the sole provider and caretaker of my two young sons—in the very situation I had tried to avoid by doing things the "right way."

This digression into my personal life and motivations for motherhood is not insignificant: my experiences helped to frame my research questions and brought me closer to my subject. Most of the women in this study were much like me: in their late twenties to early forties, educated, professional, mostly white, and struggling with the decision of how and when to conceive, raising children, or struggling with infertility. I wanted to know why some women are able to go against the social grain and venture into a form of motherhood that has been historically stigmatized in American society. How are women's self-esteem and sexuality affected by motherhood versus infertility? How do women choose a donor when they do not have to be concerned about matching the physical characteristics of a husband? How has technology opened up opportunities for women that were previously unavailable? And, on a larger scale, how does the sociopolitical climate affect access to reproductive technologies and the creation of alternative families? As I reached into these women's personal lives and decisions, my admiration for them grew. Why was it they were able to take control over their lives and choose a nonconventional way of becoming a mother but I was not?

There was another personal event that influenced my connection to this work. When I was just entering high school, a girl who had once been a friend spread a rumor around my school that I was a lesbian, even though she knew I actually had crush on her brother. One day, as I stepped off the bus and onto my front lawn, a truck full of boys from my high school pulled up, and she jumped out the back of the truck. Right in front of my house, she grabbed me by the hair, started punching me in the face and stomach, and dragged me to the ground, where she continued her assault. The boys in the truck punched their fists in the air, hurled insults at me, and cheered her on for pummeling the presumed lesbian—an affront to their masculinity?

While I had always been an empathetic child and could easily feel other people's feelings, that one incident gave me embodied experience of what it is like to be victimized for being who I am or who I am presumed to be. I suddenly felt as though I had to prove my heterosexuality—and scramble to overcome being attacked, ostracized, and marginalized—at a time when conforming to heteronormative standards felt like the only option. While that experience was certainly traumatic, it gave me a perspective I would not have otherwise had, and it was an experience I frequently flashed back to when people I interviewed told me of their struggles. I understand the violence that comes with being different—and the long-term effect it can have on someone's life, confidence, safety, and sense of well-being.

I initially conducted research for this book between 1991 and 2001, when I interviewed single women of any sexual orientation and lesbian couples. I also conducted fieldwork in several different California sperm banks and fertility clinics. In 1999 I was awarded a postdoctoral fellowship through the Social Science Research Council Sexuality Research Fellowship Program to expand the project to include sperm donor experiences and motivations. The work presented here explores the intersections between the sperm-banking industry, women who create their families with sperm donors, and the men who provide sperm for other people's families.

Much has changed since I initially conducted this research. Despite significant gains in marriage rights for same-sex couples, and significantly increased access to reproductive technologies, people forming families in the United States still face substantial challenges and threats to the security of their families. These challenges shift according to ever-fluctuating political tides. The hetero-nuclear family model is often perceived as the ideal family structure—if not the only proper family structure—in which to raise children. Yet in the trajectory of human history and across cultures, the nuclear model is a mere blip on the screen, and it is fast fading even in the United States. Same-sex couples face stigma and structural barriers to both creating their families and having access to all the protections heterosexual couples take for granted. Transgender people face even further challenges.

My children are now grown and in college. If I had not been a researcher on the infertility project at the time, I may have never been able to have them. While my path to motherhood was somewhat traditional in the sense of trying to create that "ideal" nuclear family, by raising my children on my own and being their sole provider, my experience was in many ways parallel to that of some of the single women who used a donor to create their families, but with the extra challenges that come with failed marriages and contentious separations. For a variety of reasons, including the lived reality of being a single parent struggling to support my kids, creating this book took as long as raising my sons to adulthood.

Because of that delay, however, I now have the perspective of time, allowing a broader understanding of the shifts in reproductive technologies and family creation that have occurred over a span of more than two decades. My current research on women's experiences as egg donors adds another element to my appreciation of the complex issues in third-party reproduction. This book not only situates women's experiences creating families during the onset of the so-called lesbian baby boom and the rise of groups such as Single Mothers by Choice but also ultimately explores the role of technology in the shifting landscape of family creation from the 1990s to today.

ROMANCING THE SPERM

ROMANCING THE SPERM

1 · MURPHY BROWN AND THE LESBIAN BABY BOOM

> Bearing babies irresponsibly is simply wrong.... It doesn't help matters when primetime TV has Murphy Brown, a character who supposedly epitomizes today's intelligent, highly paid professional woman, mocking the importance of fathers by bearing a child alone and calling it just another lifestyle choice.... We cannot be embarrassed out of our belief that two parents married to each other are better, in most cases, for children than one.
>
> —Vice President Dan Quayle[1]

> Societal collapse was always brought about following an advent of the deterioration of marriage and family. —Vice President Mike Pence[2]

Jackie was forty-one by the time she delivered her first child, a son, conceived via donor insemination through a Berkeley, California, sperm bank. I first met her in the fall of 1997, outside her craftsman-style duplex. She was walking up the pathway to her house, almost fifteen minutes late for our appointment, pushing a stroller. Fumbling through her diaper bag, she found her keys and opened the front door. She took her one-and-a-half-year-old out of the stroller and carried him into the house while I grabbed the stroller and parked it by the indoor stairs. She took off his tiny sweater and shoes when we got inside, and I maneuvered quickly to barely miss stepping on a rattle in the entryway. "Sorry I'm late," she said. "I was at the park with my Single Mothers by Choice group, and Logan didn't want to leave."[3] As a thirty-six-year-old single mother of two- and three-year-old sons myself at the time, in the middle of a divorce, I completely understood the challenges of leaving a park while children are playing.

Like many women her age who decide to have a child on their own, Jackie had spent years getting her education—she had a master's degree in biology—and had built a career in the health care field. As a bisexual woman, when she was in her early to mid-thirties, she had thought about having a child first in her relationship with a man, and later in her relationship with a woman using a sperm donor, and then with another woman, but none of those relationships worked out. With her son now down for a nap, she told me how she started the process to conceive her son:

When I was about a few months away from turning forty, I was really extremely depressed. My relationship was having a really rough go of it because it was becoming clear she really didn't want to be a parent—and that's what I was basing our relationship on. Then when she and I broke up, an ex-boyfriend reappeared, and he and I tried to get pregnant for a while. But that wasn't working either. I wasn't getting pregnant, and he and I broke up.

Then I was forty-one and involved with a woman again and she wanted to co-parent, but she didn't want to be pregnant. And even though we'd just met, we started looking into getting a sperm donor—an African American donor because she was African American. But she was a lot younger than me and her perception of time was different than mine, and she wanted to take more time with the process. I finally decided I was at a good point in my career, I couldn't wait to have a child at the right time in a relationship, and if I was going to do it, it had to be now. So we started at the sperm bank and got pregnant after about five tries.

Then the day I went in for my eight-week sonogram there was suddenly no heart beat. She didn't really know how to handle it, and she almost seemed relieved. So we broke up. And I kept trying on my own. I really, really didn't want to be a single parent but I didn't want to not have a child either—being a mother felt like a calling to me. And I had a good stable job with at least some maternity leave so I figured, logistically, I could do it. So after the miscarriage, the doctor put me on Perganol, a fertility drug, and after four or five more tries I got pregnant with Logan. And now I'm in the middle of trying again.

Jackie's story reflects a range of themes to be addressed throughout this book. First, facing the reality of her increasing age and declining fertility, she was aware that she only had a limited number of years left in which she would be able to have a child. Second, although she would have preferred to have a child with a partner, in the absence of being able to find an appropriate partner as ready to pursue having a family as she was—regardless of whether the partner was female or male—she decided that she would rather have a child on her own than no child at all. Third, since she had a lucrative career, good health insurance, and a good education, she could afford to support a child on her own. Jackie's story also presents a range of issues concerning how women attempt conception—whether with a male sexual partner, a known sperm donor, or an anonymous donor—and how they choose donors or the men with whom they want to have a child outside a traditional, married relationship. Jackie also, at one point, decided to use an African American donor in order to match her partner. Women have a range of reasons for why they choose the donors they choose, and these reasons may change according to whether one is conceiving on one's own or within a relationship. And finally, Jackie also experienced the trauma of numerous failed attempts at conception and pregnancy loss, before she finally delivered a healthy baby boy. She was parenting on her own when we met, and in the process of trying for a second child.

In the mid-1990s, when Jackie started her family, the sociopolitical environment surrounding what were called "alternative families" was not necessarily hospitable. While the San Francisco Bay Area has been known for its relative tolerance in terms of marital status, sexual orientation, and single parenting, stigma still existed. These prejudices emerged in terms of legal and medical policies and practices more so than in daily community life. Then-governor Pete Wilson proposed legislation to ban single men and women and same-sex couples from adopting children. His spokesperson, Sean Walsh, provided Wilson's rationale: "The Governor believes the best interest for a child is to have a mother and father in the household" (New York Times, 1996). This move took place within a broader national climate in which both the Democratic and the Republican Parties boasted of their "family values" credentials and their support for the Defense of Marriage Act, which made a ban on gay marriage federal law.

The family symbolizes the ideal relationship between the human and the natural worlds (Schneider 1968). The notion that all children need two married parents—a mother and a father—is symbolically rooted in cultural notions of "natural" procreative sex. Mary Douglas (1968) has discussed the importance of taboos in preserving the boundaries of the moral and social order, and she has analyzed the cultural anxieties that arise when "natural" categories are defied (1966, 1970). By extension, when single women or same-sex couples create families, the traditional notion of family—and compulsory heterosexuality (Rich 1980)—is challenged at a fundamental level. Motherhood among women without male partners confronts many symbolic, cultural, and political anxieties.

THE BIOPOLITICS OF FAMILY

In *The History of Sexuality*, volume 1, Michel Foucault (1980) discusses the linked notions of *biopower* and *biopolitics of the population*. *Biopower* refers to the subjugation of bodies and the control of populations through numerous and diverse techniques of the state. He states that biopower is the set of "mechanisms through which the basic biological features of the human species became the object of a political strategy, of a general strategy of power" (2007, 1). *Biopolitics*, a concept closely linked to biopower, is the social and political power over life—the link between biology and politics. These concepts are relevant to this research, and to feminist inquiries into reproduction and access to assisted reproductive technologies more broadly, because they give us insight into the linkages between cultural norms and discourses, regulatory policies, the roles of institutions, and how they affect the intimate practices of daily life. As Elizabeth Krause and Silvia De Zordo note, "The disciplining measures and related surveillance of gendered and sexual bodies aim to get people to conform to norms related to contraception and reproduction across geopolitical contexts" (2015, 7). When we look at the broader sociopolitical context in which families are created, and how different family forms are condoned (or not) in medical, legal, and political practices, we get a clearer vision of how an expanded view of what constitutes family challenges the prevailing social milieu. Not only is the regulation of family political, but so too are the individual reproductive acts of rebellion against the norm.

In the mid-1980s, when the use of conceptive technologies was relatively new but gaining in popularity, many feminist writers objected to embryological and reproductive research and technological intervention in achieving pregnancy (see, e.g., Arditti, Klein, and Minden 1984; Corea and Klein 1985; Stanworth 1987). These arguments held that such research objectifies women, exploits their pro-creativity, destroys their physical integrity, and undermines their control over their own reproduction. These critiques also included analyses of how patriarchy, race, class, gender, and power influence the position of women as consumers and patients in a local and global reproductive market (Franklin 1995, 1997; Ragone 1994; Franklin and Ragone 1998; Ginsburg and Rapp 1995; Markens 2007).

In the broad scope of reproductive politics, and the struggles over contraception, abortion, adoption, and access to reproductive technologies, ethical quandaries abound (Solinger 2013). Feminist anthropologists have had a long-standing interest in the impact of reproductive technologies on women's lives and how global inequalities are reflected in a stratified reproductive market. In *Outsourcing the Womb*, France Winddance Twine (2011) examines the dynamics of race and class in the global market for gestational surrogates. Similarly, Laura Harrison's (2016) *Brown Bodies, White Babies* explores racial differences between commissioning infertile patients and gestational surrogates, as well as how reproductive technologies are used to serve the family-creation needs of the dominant, white, heterosexual middle class. These authors provide important critiques of the reproductive industry and the role of low-income women and women of color as providers of third-party reproductive services.

The arguments against the medical and scientific control over reproduction are not as clear as they seem, however. It is true that women experiencing difficulty conceiving do become exploited consumers of modern medicine (and often "alternative" medicine as well). However, these women are also longing for a child, and if they were told by a practitioner to stop trying, they would quickly reject that doctor and seek out another who would give them more hope. Many women want, and actively seek, whatever technological means are available to them to become pregnant (Sandelowski 1993; Sargent and Bascope 1996). In *Cosmopolitan Conceptions: IVF Sojourns in Global Dubai*, Marcia Inhorn (2015) examines the stories of infertile couples who travel far and wide to get access to fertility care.

Fertility tourism, or "reprotravel," creates complex, cross-border networks and assemblages with different destinations for different reproductive purposes, including access to third-party gamete donors and gestational surrogates.

Most of the women in my study are based in the United States; however, one couple originally started their conception journey by having sperm shipped from the United States to Germany, where there were strict regulations against single women and lesbian couples having access to donor sperm. Women in my research are typically well informed about their options for treatment and recent advances in the field. They bring articles to their physicians' attention and request certain drugs and procedures. In many cases, these women research their own symptoms and conditions, diagnose their own causes of infertility, and then demand they be treated accordingly. If a woman is dissatisfied with her physician, she typically shops around until she finds one she likes.

The fact that women consider parenting without a male partner to be a viable, even preferable, alternative indicates a major shift in the constitution of the family, despite conservative rhetoric and conventional "family values." I focus specifically on single women and lesbian couples throughout this work because I am interested in how the use of technology does or does not correspond with prevailing social values and political rhetoric. The overarching questions I am asking are the following: What are the forces that influence access to reproductive technologies? How are social relations—for example, paternity, motherhood, families, and alternative kin networks—mediated through the use of technology? And how do perceptions of genetic inheritance influence donor choice? Although the users do, to a great degree, have the ability to "drive" the technology, how those technologies are used and who has access to them reflect varying philosophical and political principles. It is this manipulation of technology to achieve specific goals, according to personal and even national politics, in which I am most interested.

This ethnography takes place on three levels: (1) the daily operations of sperm banks and the business of selling sperm, (2) the individual lives of women attempting motherhood without male partners, and (3) the known and anonymous men who provide sperm to help other people have children. Looking at the junction at which these seemingly disparate entities meet provides a detailed ethnographic account of the complex interactions between technology, culture, sexuality, and lay interpretations of genetics, what I call folk genetics. Folk genetic beliefs influence how people select donors and lead to a type of "grassroots eugenics"— selecting for perceived desired traits, but in an individualized, idiosyncratic, innocuous way that is a pushback against traditional eugenics.

When I talk about "grassroots eugenics," I want to be clear that I am not referring to eugenics in the usual sense. Traditional eugenics is rooted in a racist paradigm in which some people are considered less worthy to reproduce than others. Traditional eugenics has a malevolent past. *Positive eugenics* refers to the promotion of the higher reproduction of some people over others, including fertility incentives and pronatalist policies of the state intended to increase reproduction. *Negative eugenics* includes abuses such as forced sterilization of women from specific ethnic groups, Holocaust atrocities, and the removal of children from poor people and political dissidents in order for them to be raised by "suitable" families, among other things. Grassroots eugenics can be thought of as individual reproductive rebellion against racist, sexist, and classist patriarchal models, but with the ironic twist that those doing the selecting still consider some people to be more valuable than others. The beliefs that underlie donor selection reflect a modified genetic determinism in which in addition to phenotypic traits, an array of social traits—such as donor education, hobbies, or personal likes and dislikes—are prioritized. By exploring how people choose donors, this work uncovers the social meanings embedded in genetic material.

The manipulation of reproductive technologies is consistent with perceptions of genetic fitness. Screening practices within the reproductive industry typically enhance the reproduction of certain groups of people while attempting to limit the reproduction of others. For example, many sperm banks screen out donors who do not correspond to the repository's notion of who is fit to be a genetic parent. Similar criteria can also be used to rule out potential recipients of sperm. Thus, the reproductive industry has the ability to influence what types of individuals can be reproduced and which kinds of families can be created.

The focal point of this book is how reproductive politics and notions of fitness (genetic and social) are played out through the bodies of individual women; how sperm banks act as liaisons between women and men who, otherwise, would not create a child together; and how these relationships are managed and controlled through sperm bank policies and regulations. The ways in which technologies can be manipulated to serve different interests is one point of connection between each of these areas. The uses of reproductive technologies can be simultaneously subversive and conforming, simultaneously challenging social norms on one level and reproducing them on another (Davis-Floyd and Dumit 1998, 7). Donor insemination, and reproductive technologies more broadly, facilitates alternative family arrangements within a broader sociopolitical context in which such families are regulated and stigmatized but those who have the resources to pay can find a way to get access regardless of their marital status or sexual orientation.

METHODOLOGY AND DATA

I conducted the initial phase of this research primarily in the San Francisco Bay Area over a seven-year period, between 1991 and 1998. This study includes qualitative, semistructured, open-ended interviews with women who conceived, or were attempting to conceive, with donor sperm; interviews with professionals working in the sperm-banking industry; and interviews with known and anonymous sperm bank donors. I recruited women from several sources: the larger infertility project for which I was a researcher at the time, which explored gendered emotional responses to infertility (Nachtigall, Becker, and Wozny 1992); flyers left at local sperm banks; and word of mouth.

Participants included sixteen single women of any sexual orientation and thirteen lesbian couples of reproductive age, for a total of forty-two women. Most were middle class, educated, and white. Many were Jewish, and a few were women of color. All were at various stages of trying to conceive with donor sperm. Single women were interviewed alone. Lesbian couples were first interviewed together, then independently. Interviews typically lasted two to three hours. Women who had experienced infertility often spoke longer than did those who had already conceived or delivered a child. With many of these women, I was able to conduct follow-up interviews, anywhere from six months to five years later, to find out whether any changes had occurred—such as giving birth to a child—since the first interview. Fewer than half of the women who either were not pregnant or had delivered a child at the time of the first interview had successfully conceived and delivered a child.

In 1999, with postdoctoral funding from the Social Science Research Council Sexuality Research Fellowship Program, I interviewed ten sperm donors, four of whom were known to the mothers of their children, and six of whom were anonymous donors from a sperm bank or private clinical practice. I also recruited sperm donors through flyers left at sperm banks and through personal referral. Several of the women who had children from known donors referred me to their donors to interview as well.

Aside from one phone interview with a lesbian couple in Atlanta, I conducted all of the interviews in person. The interviews were audio-recorded on tape, transcribed, and analyzed using narrative analysis. In addition to the interviews, I also conducted fieldwork in several California sperm banks and organizations offering family-building services to LGBTQ people. This fieldwork included observing daily activities, collecting de-identified donor and client profiles, attending workshops and events, and interviewing staff.

I should note that, throughout the industry, the most commonly used terms are *sperm donor* and *donation*. Men who provide sperm and women who purchase it also use these terms. *Provide* is usually a more accurate term, unless the donor is uncompensated, but it is a bit more awkward. I will use both terms throughout this book.

Compared to the rest of the United States, the San Francisco Bay Area is well known for its more liberal politics and acceptance of a range of lifestyle choices. In the 1990s, then–San Francisco mayor Willie Brown signed an ordinance allowing civil domestic partnership ceremonies and performed a number of ceremonies himself. The City of San Francisco also supported insurance coverage and other benefits for domestic partners. Single and lesbian motherhood was more common there than in other parts of the United States. There were also several sperm banks that emerged beginning around 1982 that specifically intended to provide all women "safe" alternatives to achieve pregnancy, regardless of marital status or sexual orientation.

Conducting research close to home raised some interesting theoretical and methodological questions. Laura Nader (1972) discusses the phenomenon of "studying up" and suggests anthropologists have much to contribute to an analysis of the power structures in their own society. Such an undertaking changes the "dominant-subordinate" dynamic typical in anthropological research and can affect the ways in which anthropologists build their theories. I would like to add to this the notion of "studying across"—conducting research among individuals that are very much like the researcher.

Investigations such as this further challenge the assumed distance between the self and other (Said 1978) and raise the question of how to proceed when the researcher could very easily be on the other side of the tape recorder. Indeed, my informants frequently attempted to turn the interview around and ask me to state my position as a researcher: What do I want to get out of this research? Have I published? How had I conceived my children? What was my sexual orientation? How do I plan to use my research results? How did I become interested in this subject in the first place? What are my politics? And so on. I was acutely aware throughout these queries—which I always answered honestly—that if my response to any question was not acceptable, the interview might not take place.

Many participants are professionals in the community and have, in one way or another, made a career out of donor insemination and alternative families— for example, as therapists, midwives, academics, physicians, and so on. Many are well versed in the literature on reproductive technologies, feminist theory, LGBTQ studies and queer theory, and related social science literature. Because I related to many of my informants professionally, and I was dealing with my own fertility and family-building concerns, most of my interviews were more like exchanges of information than formal interviews.

The work that follows relies heavily on "narrative ethnography"—on relaying the stories people told me regarding their experiences. Narrative analysis is widely used among anthropologists, as well as other social scientists, as narratives are viewed as a type of "cultural document" that gives "voice to bodily experience" (Becker 1999, 26). In *Writing Women's Worlds* (1993), Lila Abu-Lughod demonstrates how the use of narrative and recorded speech conveys the richness of conversations and the complexity of people's lives. The stories presented here are transcribed, edited, reorganized, and contextualized by anthropological and sociological theories and issues, combined with my own insights and experiences as a researcher in infertility and technological reproduction for over the past two decades.

AT THE INTERSECTIONS OF TECHNOLOGY, SEXUALITY, REPRODUCTION, AND GOVERNANCE

Anthropological studies of assisted reproductive technologies illustrate how they have led to fundamental changes in thinking about kinship (Strathern 1992a, 1992b; Thompson 2005; Golombok et al. 2011; Franklin and McKinnon 2001), gender (Corea 1985; Martin 1990, 1994; Inhorn 2007a; Gupta and Richters 2008; Almeling 2011), and biology (Scheper-Hughes 1985; Hubbard 1990; Martin 1991; Finkler 2000; Franklin and Ragone 1998). Techno-reproductive interventions—and who has access to them—are rooted in local and global biopolitics, mediated by gender, race, class, and sexuality (Hayden 1995; Ginsburg and Rapp 1995; Davis-Floyd and Dumit 1998; Haraway 1991). The creation of families through donor gametes— including what technologies people have access to and how they choose donors for their future children—highlights individual and cultural perceptions surrounding who has reproductive value and broader power structures in society (Yanagisako and DeLaney 1995).

This book explores intersections. When we think of intersectionality, we consider how identities of race, gender, class, ethnicity, sexual orientation, religion, mental and physical abilities, and other categories of difference and sameness in systems of oppression, domination, and discrimination interact (Crenshaw 1989). Much of the work drawing on an intersectional framework explores how these categories mutually construct one another (P. Collins 2015; P. Collins and Bilge 2016), the inequities and systemic violence imposed on black and brown bodies (D. Roberts 1998; Benjamin 2013; Ross and Solinger 2017), and the implications for reproductive justice in a world where some women's fertility, parenting rights, and reproductive power are prioritized over others (Silliman et al. 2004; Luna and Luker 2013). This framework is useful to keep in mind when we think about the medical logistics, social acceptance, and legal parameters surrounding access to family creation and recognition.

The women in my research simultaneously challenge and reflect these systems. They challenge them in that they attempted to create families outside the heteronormative nuclear family unit by having children on their own or with a female partner. They reflect the dominant systems in that the majority of the women I spoke with are upper-middle class, highly educated, white, professional women who have the financial resources to access fertility treatment, find ways to circumvent barriers that would deny them care, and pay for legal services to help them define and protect the families they create. Low-income women do not have the same access to donor sperm or fertility treatment that the women in my study had. Some women chose friends to be known donors partially due to financial constraints that prohibited them from accessing sperm from a sperm bank. When it comes to reproductive autonomy, class appears to be a determining factor in gaining access to services.

In *Invisible Families,* Mignon Moore addresses the scant attention paid to lesbian black family life, and how few scholars have made race a focus when it comes to gender, sexuality, and lesbian families, stating that "lesbian families" has become somewhat synonymous with "white middle-class lesbian families" (2011, 2). In *How to Get a Girl Pregnant,* Karleen Pendleton Jiménez chronicles her journey as a Chicana butch lesbian in Toronto trying to conceive. She notes, "In every relationship there is the potential of explosion. . . . If you have cash, you can simply buy the sperm online and avoid the risk" (2011, 8)—again pointing to how economic barriers may define the options women have on their path to pregnancy.

While my research does not specifically focus on lesbian families per se, the women who came forward to participate were predominantly white. One reason for this could be that by recruiting participants who came primarily from sperm bank and fertility clinic referrals, I unintentionally left other women out. The few women of color who did come forward found out about my research from more informal channels, such as personal referral from friends or flyers left at MAIA Midwifery, a Berkeley resource for LGBTQ family building with a holistic focus. The few women of color I did talk to did not purchase sperm from a sperm bank. Instead, they relied on their networks to help them find known donors, primarily because they wanted sperm from a donor with shared ancestry and, at the time, it was difficult to find donors of color in sperm banks.

I am also thinking about intersections in another way, reminiscent of what Nancy Scheper-Hughes and Margaret Lock refer to as the "individual body, the social body and the body politic" (1987) in their call for a critical medical anthropology. My research along this line explores the intersections between women seeking pregnancy, men providing sperm, the sperm banks and medical facilities in which sperm is provided or pregnancies occur, the ideological underpinnings of individual reproductive health providers who determine which clients they will or will not serve, and the overarching social and legal contexts governing policy around family creation and recognition.

While men and women enter into these businesses to produce and purchase a product, this is an intimate product; it enters one's body to produce a child. Sperm bank staff screen their donors, in part, according to what kinds of characteristics their clients will want, and they provide women (or other intended parents) with information about the men who will provide the products to produce their future children. Someday, perhaps eighteen years down the road, the woman or her child may actually meet the donor, and they may expand their view of family to include him in some capacity. Women using known donors may incorporate the donors into their families, albeit in a limited way.

In chapter 2, I focus on three sperm banks—although I visited more than this—that are quite divergent in their founding philosophies and reproductive policies. This is to give the reader a feel for how sperm banks conduct their business and act as liaisons between the men who provide semen and the women who receive it. It is through these sperm banks that webs of relationships are woven, creating the very fabric of women's families. It is also a marketplace where reproductive workers (donors) provide a product (semen) that is bought and sold. These connections between people—many of whom will never meet— occur because of the market for genetic material that provides "the gift of life," a child. These connections are brought about by an industry that is regulated by laws, contracts, and government. It is the manipulations of these intersections, connections, and boundaries that I find most interesting.

Chapter 3 examines how single women and lesbian couples decide to become mothers via sperm donation, how they make initial decisions about the kind of donor they want to use, how women think about parenthood, and how they experience the process of trying to conceive. Single women and lesbian couples have different challenges throughout the process. While a single woman who conceives a child through donor insemination is automatically recognized as a mother with full parental rights, lesbian couples have to bear extra expenses and overcome additional challenges to have the nonbiological mother legally recognized as the child's parent.

In chapter 4, I explore how male sexuality is regulated in the sperm bank industry and how men experience sexuality in relation to their work as sperm donors. I consider the numerous contradictions that exist in regard to semen and its collection, and how the clinical language surrounding sperm "specimens" and "deposits" reflects an uneasiness surrounding sexuality and masculinity. This chapter delves into an analysis of what semen and sperm are thought to contain—as a product, as genetic material, as a potential transmitter of medical risk, and as a contributor to a future child. Here, I explore the intersections between the different philosophical underpinnings and practices within individual sperm banks and men's experiences as sperm providers within these spaces.

Chapter 5 addresses what I call grassroots eugenics—how everyday individualistic thinking about genetic inheritance and one's reproductive values influences decisions surrounding donor selection. Donor selection is directly connected to how we think about genetic inheritance and is an expression of individually held values. When women choose sperm donors, they directly confront their own biases surrounding what kind of child they want to reproduce. The one-page sperm donor profiles provided by sperm banks construct an image of who the donor is as a person, and many women create detailed imaginings of his personality, what he looks like, what books he reads, and other personality traits. I think of sperm donor selection as a form of embodied micropolitics that reflects personal morals and values enacted through one's body, informed by one's vision of the kind of child one wants to bring into the world.

In chapter 6, we return to the sperm bank to explore how donor sperm is simultaneously conceptualized as both gift and product. As product, there are different characteristics that influence a donor's commodity value, including ancestry, his expressed motivation for becoming a donor, his willingness to have his identity released at some point in the future, and his specific medical, genetic, and social traits that may increase his popularity among potential clients. The way in which sperm donors are recruited, presented, and transacted attempts to decommodify the commodity through the language of gifts, though the exchange of sperm for money is still a business transaction. Here, I demonstrate how perceived donor altruism—a trait women look for when they choose a donor—enhances the commodity value of a donor and his sperm.

For many women, attempting to conceive a child can be a long, arduous, costly, and ultimately devastating process. In chapter 7, I explore how women experience the emotional and physical terrains of infertility. In the 1990s and early 2000s, the medical establishment and insurers saw a distinction between "medical infertility" and "social infertility." Medical infertility was defined along the heteronormative lines of inability to conceive after a year or more of trying through unprotected, heterosexual sex, and many insurers would cover some treatment and medical providers would treat their medically infertile patients. For women suffering from "social infertility"—or not having natural access to sperm—coverage and medical care were inconsistent. When women were paying hundreds of dollars a month for donor sperm and still not getting pregnant, these costs and the emotional toil added up. In this chapter, I discuss women's phenomenological experience with infertility and how it affects identity and feelings of failure.

Chapter 8 considers the question, What's alternative about family? The term *alternative* has often been used to describe LGBTQ families specifically, more so than single-parent families, or even families that are recombined through divorce and remarriage. Here, I problematize the notions of "alternative" and "traditional" and instead look toward a range of family forms in which the heterosexual nuclear model is but one of many possibilities for creating and defining family. In this chapter, I highlight different family forms and ask, How do women tell others about their decision to have a child without a male partner? What does day-to-day family life look like for single mothers and lesbian couples? And how do known donors take on redefined roles as "donor dads" and "honorary uncles"—not quite donors, but not quite fathers, either?

There have been significant changes in family formation and recognition from the 1990s to today. Through new interviews conducted in 2017, chapter 9 addresses some of those changes. Social acceptance of same-sex partners and single-parent families has increased. There is improved awareness about transgender identities and reproductive needs, and language has evolved to reflect these changes. Medical technologies and access to reproductive technologies and fertility treatment have expanded dramatically, including a range of options available for single people and same-sex couples who can afford it. The U.S. Supreme Court's *Obergefell v. Hodges* decision recognized the right of same-sex couples to marry. However, same-sex married couples still face obstacles to their legal rights as parents to children born into those unions, but that too appears to be changing. While there have been significant advances, there are also significant continuing challenges for those who do not fit into the heterosexual, married, nuclear image of family—especially on the ever-fluctuating political front.

Ultimately, this work explores how social forces influence the use of technology. When the technology is connected to sexuality and reproduction, public tensions become more evident. Throughout history, sexuality and reproduction have been subject to various forms of state control, from positive and negative eugenic policies, to laws governing adoption and custody. The shifting use of reproductive technologies points to a new order for the production of life, nature, and the body through biologically based interventions—what Paul Rabinow (1992) has called "biosociality."

Policies surrounding the use of these technologies vary among individual clinics and according to geographic location, and they are embedded in cultural discourses of sexuality, normalcy, and "family values." This book focuses on the uses of technology and cultural meanings surrounding genetics, reproduction, and the family at four intersecting levels: (1) women seeking motherhood, (2) men providing sperm, (3) the reproductive and sperm-banking industries, and (4) the shifting regulatory landscape surrounding reproductive politics and policies. Brought together, we see how these interconnections simultaneously reflect, reinforce, and challenge prevailing social conventions and illuminate areas of conformity, resistance, and agency. Of primary import are the complex interactions between technology, culture, and sexuality in what has been one of the most contested arenas of public debate—the creation of (alternative) families.

Technology enables the separation of sexual intercourse and reproduction, yet intimate connections remain. Sperm is a product that can be bought and sold, but it comes from people—people who have lives of their own, who may think about the children their sperm produced and the mothers who raised them. Women who purchase or use donor sperm to have children think about the men who provide it—whether they ever actually meet or not. Some of these thoughts include fantasies or ideas about what their child's donor looks like, what he acts like, or who he is in the world. Donor-conceived children, too, may be curious, may also have fantasies about their donors, and may wonder whether they have his eyes, his smile, or his quirky sense of humor. In these largely technological, asensual spaces, "romancing"—the process of embellishing something into a romantic ideal—still exists, and sperm is at the heart of it. This book sheds light on these detached human connections in simultaneously personal and depersonalized spaces.

2 · TECHNOLOGIES AND POLITICS OF REPRODUCTION

> One thing that I find very interesting is the strong influence on how technology gets presented in our society as the people who are using it. Our approach is, you pay attention to your users and they're going to drive the technology. —Barbara Raboy, co-founder, The Sperm Bank of California

Advances in reproductive technologies occur at such a rapid pace that it is nearly impossible to address the social, legal, and ethical challenges before they are integrated into medical practice. Assisted reproductive technologies have led to rapid changes in the meaning of personhood, parenthood, kinship, family, and gender—as well as a separation of heterosexual sex and procreation—pushing the limits of biology (Strathern 1992b). It is now possible for a couple to give birth to a child created entirely from donor gametes who has absolutely no biological link to either parent. Postmenopausal women can carry and deliver children—their own grandchildren—for their daughters. A woman can become impregnated with her partner's sperm after his death. A woman who is clinically brain-dead can be sustained on life support to bring an infant to full term. A fetus can receive surgery and be delivered months later. Women are now freezing eggs to delay childbearing. While users drive technology, we as a society are also transformed by it.

Discourse on genetics and reproductive technologies poses challenges to anthropology. Applications of these forms of science go to the heart of prevailing ethical dilemmas and yield insights into the value of the nuclear family, as well as of the primacy of biological over any other kind of parenthood. How reproductive technologies are accessed and utilized provides insight into how we think about genetics, culture, and power. Power is manifest at different levels of society, revealing the competing discourses of church, state, medicine, and feminism in Euro-American societies and across the globe. Research on genetic and reproductive technologies challenges the division of natural and social and moves anthropology to a more fertile ground—one in which the interplays between culture and biology are revealed, beyond the boundaries of nature-versus-nurture debates.

In the United States, when the sperm bank and reproductive technology industries were first getting their start, there was a lack of uniform regulations regarding who was eligible for insemination or treatment for infertility. Some individual sperm banks and private physicians made their own policies regarding to whom they would provide these services. Although there were sperm banks and physicians that helped single women and lesbian couples conceive, many banks and reproductive clinics had explicit policies to provide treatment only to heterosexual (usually married) couples. Some sperm banks emerged specifically to reach a neglected population—single women and lesbian couples—and were able to build a substantial international clientele.

Internationally, the regulation of donor insemination, and the climate of acceptance surrounding donor insemination for single women and lesbian couples, varied. These restrictions also changed over time. When I first started this research in the 1990s, most European countries had severe restrictions prohibiting single women and lesbian couples from having access to donor sperm. Some of these policies have changed in the past thirty years, but, surprisingly, most have not. In 1990 Great Britain had one of the most restrictive policies, denying access to donor insemination and infertility treatment for single women and lesbian couples. These restrictions were based on the notion that children need a father.[1] The United Kingdom changed this policy in 2008.[2] Table 2.1 demonstrates different international laws surrounding access to donor insemination in the 1990s. Since 1997, only Sweden, the United Kingdom, and Finland have changed their regulations to allow donor insemination for single women and lesbian couples.

Aside from the issue of access, regulations also vary with respect to whether donor compensation is permitted, as well as whether donor identity release is required or optional. These country-specific regulations reflect different cultural, ethical, and moral sensibilities.

In the 1990s only a handful of western European countries permitted single women and lesbians access to donor insemination. In some countries where donor insemination was not officially available, some women were able to find a private physician willing to help them conceive. Others had sperm shipped from abroad— initially the United States, and later Denmark—for self-insemination. In some countries, however, strict guidelines prohibited private doctors from performing inseminations, lest they be prosecuted. Women may still have had the option of entering into private arrangements with known donors and inseminating at home; however, these arrangements can also be risky, especially where child custody is an issue. Until 2005, a Swedish woman who was inseminated with donor sperm could face legal problems, for Swedish law stated a child must have a known father (Berggren 1997, 208). Out of the thirteen countries listed in table 2.1, only Finland

TABLE 2.1   Legal access to donor insemination for single women and lesbian couples in western Europe

Country	Lesbians	Single women	Public access	Private access	Strict regulations
Austria	No	No	No	Limited	Yes
Belgium	Yes	Yes	No	Limited	Yes
Finland[a]	No	No	No	Limited	No, but guidelines against
France	No	No	No	Very limited	Yes
Germany	No	No	No	Very limited	Yes—can be prosecuted
Ireland	Limited	Limited	One public clinic	Yes	No
Italy	No	No	No	No—penalties to doctors	Yes
Netherlands	Yes	Yes	Yes	Yes	No
Norway	Yes	Yes	Yes	Yes	No
Spain	Yes	Yes	Yes	Yes	no
Sweden[a]	No	No	No	No	Yes
Switzerland	Yes	Yes	Variable	Variable	No
United Kingdom[a]	No	No	No	No	Yes

SOURCE: Adapted from Griffin and Mulholland (1997).
[a] Indicates countries where policies have changed since 1997, now permitting access to donor sperm for single women and lesbian couples.

(in 2007), Sweden (for lesbian couples in 2005 and single women in 2016), and the United Kingdom (in 2008) changed their policies to allow access for single women and lesbian couples. Spain has had among the most progressive policies regarding access to donor sperm and infertility treatment for single women and lesbian couples; however, in Spain, donor anonymity is required. Currently, while egg, sperm, and embryo donation are permitted in Spain, surrogacy is not allowed under Spanish law, as the woman who gives birth to a child is legally recognized as the mother.

In countries where donor insemination is highly regulated as a matter of national policy, the issues of social engineering and the meaning of family becomes much more explicit (Shore 1992). Many of the debates surrounding limiting access to donor insemination to heterosexual married couples assume the child's right to have a known father. Indeed, according to the 1991 Child Support Act in the

United Kingdom, a man who acts as a semen donor can be held liable for providing support for any children born of his donated sperm (Donovan 1997, 221). Hence, potential donors in Great Britain might be more reluctant to help a woman conceive a child on her own.

There are many social and political implications surrounding who has access to treatment. The high cost of reproductive technologies poses economic barriers to lower-income people seeking access to services and reflects social stratification along the lines of race and class. Screening policies can also prioritize the creation of some families over others, weeding out potential clients who do not reflect the clinic's image of the "ideal" family. Limited access to reproductive technologies points to how family is socially, politically, legally, medically, and morally constructed, and how some families are valued over others.

Social studies of science and technology and feminist critiques of science demonstrate the linkages between knowledge and culture (Keller 1985; Latour and Woolgar 1986; Nader 1996). Clifford Geertz (1973), for example, suggests that cultural systems can best be understood in terms of their capacity to express the nature of the world and to shape the world to their dimensions. Anthropologists of science attempt to demonstrate how scientific practices develop in relation to social concerns, as well as the relations of power in the production and utilization of science both locally and globally (Flower and Heath 1993; Forsythe 1992; Hess 1992; Layne 1992; Rabinow 1993). Medical anthropologists, in particular, have challenged the facticity of biomedical knowledge—recognizing that both knowledge and practice are culturally constructed (Franklin 1995; Lock and Gordon 1988; Lock and Lindenbaum 1993).

Technological advances have also been analyzed as a reflection of the established social environment of corporate capitalism (Noble 1977; Hubbard and Wald 1993) that operates within and reinforces pre-existing social inequalities (Duster 1990; Wajcman 1991). The management of biological reproduction has been viewed as a mechanism of social reproduction (Morsy 1990; Rapp 1988), where the medical and technological treatment of infertility confirms the racial, class-based, and social prejudices of our society (Mosher and Pratt 1982). Thinking about assisted reproductive technologies, who has access to treatment, how donors are chosen, and how family is defined gives us insight into the nexus of cultural values and how those values are reproduced through individual bodies.

Differential access to procedures like in vitro fertilization, affected by economic as well as social constraints, seems to reflect the dominant concern in our society for the "ideal" child, as well as for the "proper" parental unit. Clearly, this connection between social biases and reproduction is central to this research. Technologies—like rules—can be manipulated to meet individual needs. Thus, the "moral order of society" is not always maintained according to the predominant ideologies but rather is negotiated at the individual level, through individual agency.

HISTORICAL BACKGROUND TO DONOR INSEMINATION

The first reported incident of the use of donor sperm for insemination in the United States was in 1884 (Small and Turksoy 1985). By 1924, 123 cases of human donor insemination were reported, resulting in forty-seven pregnancies (Rohleder 1934). It has been estimated that between one thousand and seven thousand inseminations were performed using donor sperm between 1950 and 1960, although the number of live births is not indicated (Golin 1962; Schellan 1957). In the late 1980s and early 1990s, by most estimates there were approximately twenty-three thousand to thirty thousand donor inseminations per year that resulted in live births (Shapiro and Schultz 1990; U.S. Congress, Office of Technology Assessment, 1988). A 1996 study of thirty-one sperm banks found that, although single women and lesbian couples are represented among sperm recipients at some banks, the majority of clients nationwide are heterosexual married couples (Hanson 1996). However, estimates are inaccurate. And there is still no reliable tracking of how many donor-conceived children are born per year. In addition, intracytoplasmic sperm injection—which enables a single sperm to be injected directly into an egg—offered heterosexual couples other alternatives for using the partner's sperm. This reduced their need for sperm donors. The demand for sperm donors among women without male partners remained the same or intensified.

Since the 1970s, self-insemination using a known donor emerged in direct response to screening procedures within the medical establishment that limited access for unmarried women. In fact, numerous self-help works were published on this procedure (Feminist Self-Insemination Group 1980; Hornstein 1984; Klein 1984; Stern 1980; Wolf 1982). It has been estimated that by 1980, 1,500 unmarried women gave birth to children as a result of donor insemination (Fleming 1980). It is unknown how many children were conceived through self-insemination. The majority of the impetus for the self-insemination movement came from lesbian women, demonstrating the political nature of reproductive control. Self-insemination emerged in direct response to screening procedures within the medical establishment, which traditionally limited access for unmarried women. Lesbian self-insemination challenged power structures, traditional discourses of family, and "modes of procreation" (Agigian 2004).

Limited access to donor sperm also prompted the emergence of sperm banks that openly catered to single women and lesbian couples. In 1982, founders of a feminist women's health center in Oakland, California, launched the first sperm bank—The Sperm Bank of California—that openly provided donor sperm to anyone who needed it to create a family, including unmarried women and lesbian couples. The Sperm Bank of California (TSBC), then directed by Barbara Raboy, was also the first sperm bank to offer donor-identity release, so donor-conceived children could connect with their donors when they reached the age of eighteen. With the rise of HIV/AIDS, purchasing semen from a sperm bank became increasingly more popular than self-insemination with a known donor (usually a friend or acquaintance of the woman who wished to conceive). Medical screening and a six-month quarantine of donor semen samples made frozen donor semen from sperm banks safer than semen from a known donor.

In the 1990s in United States, legislation regarding access to donor sperm varied from state to state. The majority of legislation appeared to deny nonmarried women access to donor sperm (Pilpel 1985; Polakow 1993); but others interpret legislation in terms of its permission of access (Kritchevsky 1981). Only Oregon explicitly allowed the use of donor insemination by nonmarried women ("Reproductive Technology" 1985; Pilpel 1985).

In the United Kingdom, Robert Snowden, Geoffrey Duncan Mitchell, and E. M. Snowden (1983) analyzed cases of couples who had utilized donor insemination to become pregnant. Their research recommended two policies: one, parents who use donor insemination should disclose the nature of conception to their offspring, and two, lesbians and single women should not have access. In 1984 in the United Kingdom, the Warnock Committee attempted to regulate how such technologies should be used. They assumed the country as a whole shared certain ideas about the family that could be discovered and implemented in policies governing reproductive technologies (Cannell 1990). Their task was to produce a moral consensus that effectively dealt with conflicting religious and cultural attitudes. They also recommended policies prohibiting unmarried women access to donor insemination and other reproductive technologies.

The issue of access to reproductive technologies demonstrates culturally held notions of who is fit to become a parent according to heteronormative perceptions of family. Policies governing technological reproduction are embedded in a long history of scientific and lay notions regarding biological inheritance and parental fitness. Young unmarried mothers—especially those who are poor and without a college education or professional career—face enormous stigma (Edin and Kefalas 2011). Women who choose to pay for donor sperm, however, are rarely poor, and most face a different challenge: by putting their education and careers first over motherhood, many have reached the age at which conception becomes more difficult.

Increasing use of donor insemination as a method of conception merits a close examination of the impact such technologies have on broader cultural and political meanings of family. The ways in which the use of donor insemination and other reproductive technologies are negotiated and legislated provide insight into the complex controversies regarding sexuality, reproduction, and parenthood in advanced capitalist societies (Stanworth 1987, 18). Sperm bank businesses emerged in response to these social constraints, which both reconfirm and challenge the status quo.

Individual sperm bank policies directly correspond to the individual philosophies of the people who found them. Policies about who a repository accepts as a client or a donor are by no means uniform throughout the industry. In fact, what makes an acceptable donor or recipient is often based as much on divergent social screening processes as on any exclusionary criteria grounded in scientific or medical "facts." These policies can be a means of implementing social engineering under the guise of medical authority. Many in vitro fertilization programs and sperm banks have screening procedures that weed out unmarried couples and single women. For example, one sperm bank, the Repository for Germinal Choice (RGC), only accepts married women under age thirty-eight who are free of any genetic abnormalities, who have the written consent of their husbands, and who have met the repository's criteria for high intelligence. Here, individual values surrounding family, combined with a positive eugenic program, are reproduced through the sperm bank's policies and exclusionary practices.

In the San Francisco Bay Area in the 1990s, several sperm banks and a few fertility clinics accepted single and lesbian women for treatment. TSBC in Berkeley was founded on the premise of offering services to all women, regardless of marital status or sexual orientation. Rainbow Flag Health Services (RFHS), in Oakland, California, specifically served the LGBTQ community by having almost exclusively gay donors and bisexual and lesbian clients. In the absence of uniform standards for screening, technology-assisted reproduction has largely been driven by the screening policies of individual sperm banks and reproductive clinics, with a great deal of variation.

SPERM BANK PHILOSOPHIES AND DAILY PRACTICE

I conducted fieldwork at RGC, RFHS, and TSBC, spending the most time at TSBC. Each of these sperm banks was founded according to different philosophies and principles that affected their reproductive practices, including how donors were screened and selected, what categories of clients they served, perceptions of medical and social risk, and other factors. At TSBC, I attended meetings and support groups and collected extensive data from their files. The underlying philosophies and goals of these different sperm banks reflect different, often conflicting, missions related to sexuality, reproduction, and, to some degree, social engineering.

Genius Sperm and Social Engineering

> Our philosophy was we wanted the best and the brightest ... so that we can give children the best possible start in life.   —Anita Neff, RGC

Hermann Muller, an American geneticist, calculated what he considered to be the amount of genetic load (i.e., deleterious genes) the human race as a whole could accommodate, and he postulated how human evolution could be guided and improved through selective reproduction (1959, 1962). He expected that people with high genetic loads would voluntarily refrain from procreation out of a sense of civic duty. Similarly, it would be considered "a social service for those more fortunately endowed to reproduce more than the average extent" (Muller 1950 150). Muller thus presented a method to help offset the effects of increased genetic load—utilizing recent developments in the field of artificial insemination. He proposed that an individual's sperm could be frozen, and that after the death of the donor—when it could be determined that the individual had truly led an exceptional life—the sperm could be thawed and used to inseminate a healthy and intelligent female recipient. This was seen as an effort to help guide humankind's evolution to the highest standard possible.

In the early 1960s Muller, with the encouragement of many of his colleagues, was considering establishing a sperm bank to increase the reproduction of people who met his criteria for genetic fitness. Robert K. Graham shared his mission and offered to fund the project—at the tune of $300,000 a year—to maintain the sperm of exceptional men in a liquid-nitrogen repository. The primary criteria used for donor selection were high levels of altruism and intelligence. Muller proposed that Julian Huxley would be a good candidate, and Graham suggested that Muller would be an ideal donor. Muller finally abandoned the project, reportedly because he felt Graham put too much emphasis on intelligence and too little on altruism (Kevles 1985). Muller died in 1967.

There was a great deal of support for this project among evolutionists, including Ernst Mayr, Francis Crick, and Aldous Huxley, who saw this as an improvement over earlier eugenic schemes to sterilize "genetic inferiors." William Shockley, a physicist, Nobel Prize winner, and extensive writer on dysgenics and population, was a donor at this repository at the age of seventy. The assumption is that intelligence and altruism are heritable traits, and that by permitting a few gifted men to produce more offspring than they would normally, they could positively affect the human gene pool. Like Muller, Graham wrote extensively about his views on improving the human gene pool through donor insemination; see his *The Future of Man* (1970), and other materials.

In 1980, well after Muller's death, Graham created the Hermann J. Muller Repository for Germinal Choice, housed in Escondido, California (Plotz 2005). Initially, the sperm stored there came exclusively from Nobel laureate donors, who were almost exclusively white, married, heterosexual men. This criterion was later relaxed to include the sperm of other scientists, and even one Olympic athlete. The bank later relaxed its standards even more to include "men in excellent health who in addition . . . demonstrate great potential." Its purpose was to "put more genes from some of our best men into the human gene pool" and to "give babies the best possible start in life."

The initial costs at this bank for intended parents wishing to purchase sperm included a $100 application fee, a $200 cryogenic tank fee, and a $3,000 program fee. The monthly cost was approximately $550, or $183 per vial of semen—slightly more expensive than most other banks, which charged between $100 and $140 per vial of semen. These fees included three vials of semen per month for up to six months.

This sperm bank explicitly did not serve single women and lesbians, so I did not recruit research subjects from this site. In an interview with the clinic's director in 1998, I learned most of its clients were physicians and their wives. During the first few years of operation at RGC, a single woman lied about her marital status and conceived a child using their donor sperm. This outraged Graham, and he created stricter controls to ensure this would not happen again. After this incident, he required each client to provide copies of her marriage license and driver's license, a signed and notarized consent form giving the husband's consent, and a letter written by a physician stating that he or she had treated the couple for infertility and would assist with the inseminations.

Because unmarried women were specifically excluded from being served by RGC, I wanted to know more about the bank's underlying assumptions surrounding parental fitness and meanings of family that influenced its mission and practice. What did its staff mean by the "best possible start in life"? What were their assumptions surrounding genetic inheritance? How do these perspectives influence who they chose as donors and recipients? To some degree, their restrictive policies represented the broader context of U.S. mainstream conservative culture at the time, found outside the relatively progressive San Francisco Bay Area.

I first made an appointment to interview Graham in 1996. This was a bit ambitious, as I had just delivered my second child, had another son under two, and was having difficulties in my marriage. Circumstances prohibited me from making the trek from Berkeley down to Escondido. About a year later, when I called to reschedule, Graham had already passed away. He was ninety-one and died after a fall in his hotel bathtub. As a newly divorced single mother of two toddlers, I asked my parents to watch my sons so I could travel to Escondido for the interview with the director of RGC. I met Anita Neff in 1998. She had been the administrative director of RGC since before Graham's death.

I drove up and parked at the unassuming Escondido office building, which had tinted glass doors. "This can't possibly be the right place," I thought. It did not look anything like any of the other sperm banks I had been to. The barely noticeable sign by the door told me otherwise. I opened the door and walked in. Anita sat at the front desk, prepared for my arrival. Since she was not the founder, but rather an employee, her personal philosophies regarding reproduction were not completely in line with the founding and operating principles of the repository. Yet she was still well versed in what those principles were. The following is Anita's understanding of how the repository was founded and developed: "Dr. Graham and Dr. Muller came up with the concept in 1963, I think it was when they signed the agreement that they would do this [start the repository]. Then in the late seventies, early eighties, they opened the doors. Actually, Dr. Graham opened the doors; Muller had died by then. The first child was born in 1982, and we currently have 222 offspring from our program. Dr. Graham just died a year ago at ninety-one, and he actively ran it until then."

Anita led me down the hallway to the back office as she talked. As we walked, I glanced at the walls and noticed photograph after photograph of blond-haired, mostly blue-eyed children. There was one particularly large photograph of a blond-haired boy of about ten, dressed in a light suit and staring directly at me. I wondered why his photograph held such prominence over the others. Some of the kids were clearly biologically related. Although there was nothing sinister about these children in and of themselves, the combination of almost twenty portraits of fair-haired children in this single space was jarring. The walls displayed a visual representation of the repository's eugenic mission.

I asked Anita about how they recruit and select their donors. "They started out with the concept that they wanted the best and the brightest and they thought Nobel laureates would best fit that category." She continued,

> In order to find donors we use *Who's Who* and we look for people who graduated at the top of their class, or who have patents pending, or anything that makes them outstanding. We look through magazines, newspapers, articles, anything. Then we write them. Usually, it's men in the sciences, because that was Dr. Graham's background. But we really want to see they are achieving or excelling above other people—we just know they're high achieving and exceptional men. We also use criteria from the Mensa list for people who would qualify to belong to that society in order to become donors.
>
> Health is obviously the main criteria, but after health comes IQ and their ability to function in society. We have turned down men that were very, very smart and healthy, but they were the kind of people who were not very productive in society, it was like they just sat around and thought all day. And we try to get more well-rounded people because we need productive people in the world who can interact and have a social life—we need people, not robots. It is this kind of man— that is exceptional and altruistic—that our repository seeks.

At RGC there are numerous assumptions regarding what it means to give a child "the best possible start in life." These assumptions are based both on speculative theories of genetic inheritance and on the premise that in order to be healthy and well socialized, all children need to grow up in a family in which there are two parents who are married and heterosexual. At the genetic level, RGC assumes that great health, high IQ, and high achievement can all be passed down from donor to offspring. Creating productive, smart, exceptional, and altruistic people who have a social life is a primary goal for this repository. For a repository so focused on "science," it is bewildering that its staff perceive a certain personality type— for example, someone smart who does more than sit around thinking all day—as genetically predetermined, especially in the absence of any scientific data to support this level of genetic determinism.

Another goal of this sperm bank is to positively affect the human gene pool. As Graham states in RGC's promotional materials,

> With bright mothers and genius [donor] fathers the probability of bright, healthy and creative children is maximized. Even if none of these children prove to be geniuses, they still represent an enrichment of the human gene pool; a wider distribution of genes for high intelligence than would have taken place otherwise. . . . If there were hundreds of banks, at least one in each city of size, this could result in thousands of bright, useful citizens who otherwise would not have been born or probably would not be as intelligent. Now, in this century, the new science of genetics has powerfully reinforced man's ability to transcend himself and thus to reach new heights of competence.

RGC clearly was founded as a program promoting positive eugenics. The heritability of certain desirable traits—such as intelligence, altruism, and high accomplishment—is tenuous or, at best, unproved. The assumptions and values surrounding reproduction and the family are usually consistent between clients and the sperm banks they choose.

In one of my earliest interviews with heterosexual couples using donor sperm, one couple had gone to what they called the "genius sperm bank" in hopes of finding an intelligent donor. When I asked them why they did not use a local sperm bank, they explained, "The best sperm we could find at the local bank was that of a Russian cashier. I don't know how much of intelligence is inherited or environmental, but I'd rather have my kid have the best chance of becoming a scientist if they want to, rather than having to go through life as a cashier or something." In this couple's opinion, a child's potential was directly linked to the potential of the sperm donor. These people wanted an "intelligent" child and therefore contracted with the sperm bank they thought was most likely to give them what they wanted.

Building LGBTQ Communities through Donor Insemination

Housed in an old Victorian building in Oakland, RFHS was founded in 1995.[3] It specifically served the LGBTQ community, had completely open policies regarding releasing the donor's identity to the mother when the offspring reached three months old, and required contact between the donor and his offspring. Incidentally, RFHS opposed male circumcision and thus required that any male children born not be circumcised. According to Leland Traiman, a gay male and RFHS' founder, the bank's goal was to build a stronger lesbian and gay community by assisting lesbians and gay men to bring children into their families. Of the fifteen women he had as clients at the time of this fieldwork, only one of them was heterosexual; of the eighteen or so donors, two of them were heterosexual and one was bisexual. The rest were gay.

Leland was going about his work as we talked, counting the number of sperm in a sample under a microscope. I followed him around with my tape recorder asking questions.

I knew a lot of women who were around the age of forty, and they went to the sperm bank and they felt bad about going to the sperm bank because they wanted to know who the guy was. Well, the sperm bank wasn't very satisfying. They would never find out who the donor is, or maybe the kid would find out when the kid is eighteen. They wanted another alternative. So I thought, let's start a sperm bank where we tell the recipients who the donor is when the child is three months old. Then, the more and more I got into it, I realized that the two other sperm banks in the Bay Area [, which] were founded by lesbians and run by lesbians, don't accept gay men as donors. So, I'm the only show in town in terms of accepting gay men as donors.

Right when I turned thirty, I was trying to figure out how I could have kids and then, shortly after that, in 1982, was when the AIDS epidemic started. We didn't know who was infected and who wasn't and so it just didn't seem like a wise idea to have kids.

I see what I do as extremely political and it's only political because of the opposition. Essentially, it is people who just want families and it becomes political because of bigotry. Is praying in a synagogue political? Well, it certainly was in Germany in the thirties. But generally we don't think it is. So, what I'm doing is political, but only because of the bigoted atmosphere surrounding me.

So I said to myself, "I'm forty. I'm sick and tired of working for other people. I don't like the way the present sperm banks are running their operations." I thought, "I'm a nurse practitioner. I can do this."

Leland's motivations emerged from his own frustration of "chasing parenthood" for most of his adult life, and from the fact that he felt gay males were discriminated against at other banks. Assisting lesbians and gay men to bring children into their families directly connects the policies of the sperm repository to his personal situation of wanting children and his political stance—wanting to help strengthen the lesbian and gay community. Both of these interests are connected to his policy of donor identity release when the child reaches three months of age. His intention is to strengthen the connections between offspring and donor parent by providing early contact and the potential for building a relationship. This policy also establishes contact between lesbian mothers and the donor of their offspring, with the expectation that they will have an amicable relationship and the child will be permitted some contact with the donor—even though the donor has no legal rights and is not considered the legal father.

Reproductive Choice and Women's Empowerment

TSBC, originally located in Oakland, was founded in 1982 and was initially part of the Oakland Feminist Women's Health Center. The women's health collective saw a need to make sperm available to all women, and was the first to cater specifically to single women and lesbians, as well as to offer donor-identity release. The term *identity release* ® is used by TSBC to refer to the process by which donors agree to have their identity released to any child born from their sperm when the child reaches eighteen. Throughout the industry, in other sperm banks the term *open identity* is often used to describe the same thing. TSBC's mission is to "challenge fundamental prejudices and exclusionary policies of the sperm banking and medical communities" (The Sperm Bank of California 1991, 2). It was founded on the principle of "reproductive freedom for all individuals regardless of marital status, sexual preferences, age, race, or religion" (The Sperm Bank of California 1991). In the 1990s, initial fees included a $400 application fee, plus approximately $108 per vial of semen. In 1988 TSBC had split off from the Oakland Feminist Women's Health Center to incorporate as an independent nonprofit corporation, the Sperm Bank of California Reproductive Technologies Inc.

I originally interviewed Barbara Raboy, co-founder and director of TSBC, in 1991, when the bank was housed in an old Victorian-style building in Oakland. With hardwood floors and an inviting lavender décor, it had the friendly flair of a community women's clinic. In 1995 the bank moved to a relatively new office building in downtown Berkeley, with a buzzer for entry. Its new location had a much more clinical feel, with more distinct offices and private rooms where women waited to pick up their orders.

Donors and recipients did not usually come into contact with one another. Donors entered through the back door, and recipients entered through the front. Before TSBC moved to an office that provided a spatial arrangement separating donors from recipients, they were generally separated by time—donors and recipients were scheduled for appointments at different times in order to preserve anonymity. When a woman arrived for a pickup of reserved semen, she was typically asked to wait in one of the waiting rooms until one of the clinic's workers could retrieve her vial and the portable liquid nitrogen tank that keeps the sperm frozen until it is ready to be thawed for insemination.

This sperm bank also provided monthly support groups where women could come to hear a speaker talk about a specific aspect of donor insemination. Women did come into contact with one another on these occasions, so some recipients were not anonymous to one another, though participation in the support groups was optional. Some of them were TSBC clients, and some of them were considering it. I spent a great deal of time there collecting data from files, interviewing office staff, attending support groups, and observing daily operations. I recruited many of my informants from this site through flyers and the TSBC newsletter.

TSBC is open to anyone who wants to purchase sperm in order to achieve a pregnancy, although the majority of the clients are single women or lesbian couples; less than a third are heterosexual couples. Barbara tells the story of how the sperm bank got started:

We were originally a women's clinic providing medical services. We performed abortions and taught about birth control methods, and I had been one of the fertility instructors, teaching women how to avoid pregnancies. I had noticed over the months that women called and asked about how to become pregnant. So we decided to start a pregnancy facility. We decided that we really needed to provide a supportive environment for women. So, in the summer of 1982, I got the OK to start and keep a donor study. There were doctors in the Bay Area doing inseminations with donor sperm. Some were using fresh semen, and some were getting it directly from sperm banks. I visited another women's clinic in Southern California because I had heard they had this "self-help" donor insemination program. I looked at some other programs as prototypes and came up with a proposal for starting a sperm bank up here—a woman-controlled sperm bank.

One of the things I am most proud of is that here, we give access to single women—that isn't always the case at other banks. I didn't want to have a sperm bank if I couldn't offer the services to everyone. But that was very difficult for many people in the medical profession to swallow because there was a lot of stigma attached to women having children on their own. Many of these banks and clinics, you know, you don't have to read their brochures very far to know what their politics are. Usually, what they don't tell you is much more to the point than what they do mention. A lot of what these banks were doing served the medical community and the doctors would get the sperm and put it into their patients, so there was no direct link between the recipient of that semen and the sperm bank. It was up to the doctor to determine who he would or would not inseminate. And most doctors would only serve heterosexual married couples.

So, we kind of shook up the sperm bank community. For the first four or five years, people were just struggling because, there we were, knowing the technology—and not being scientists—but being scientific about it. But we were really strong in our politics, and I think what we really did, which is probably the greatest contribution for the sperm bank, is just to lay that out on the table. We sort of popularized the concept of a "sperm bank." I think now the stigma has decreased somewhat because of our operation.

TSBC emphasized the importance of women helping themselves—teaching them how to take responsibility for their own bodies and offering reproductive choices. This focus on helping women to empower themselves, with an emphasis on enhancing reproductive options for all women, proved to be a major impetus to the creation of this repository. Although this practice is now much more clinical than it was in 1991, when I first interviewed Barbara, there was still a strong emphasis on the relationships that are created through the repository—with both the women and the donors. It is this political philosophy that women, regardless of their marital status or sexual orientation, should be provided with safe options for creating their families that Barbara worked to maintain in her practice.

Barbara also addressed the connection between politics, science, and access to technology. For her, to have a woman-oriented practice that emphasizes reproductive choice and self-empowerment through technology is political. By offering services to women, regardless of marital status or sexual orientation, she confronted a medical community that typically offered reproductive services only to married, heterosexual women. Her practice has played a pivotal role in the reproductive industry by offering services to single women, but also by destigmatizing pregnancy out of wedlock and popularizing the notion of the "sperm bank"—taking the sale of sperm out of the sole domain of private doctors and offering it on a larger scale.

She also addressed how users drive technology. This is an important point. Technology is not created in a social vacuum. Reproductive technologies, including artificial insemination, were originally intended for heterosexual, married couples. However, since male-factor infertility is only responsible for approximately one-third of all infertility in heterosexual couples, there is a much larger client base when sperm can be sold to women who do not normally have access to it. The so-called lesbian baby boom in the San Francisco Bay Area is largely attributable to the sperm bank industry. A technology originally intended for use by one group of people has been accessed by others and has allowed for the construction of new family forms.

CONCLUSION

Each of the sperm banks discussed in this chapter was established according to its founders' personal convictions about human reproduction, and each broadened the definition of family. They decided who would become a donor and who would become a client. Whether it is providing access and choices to all women, building stronger lesbian and gay communities, or promoting the reproduction of the world's most "exceptional" men, the policies of each of these three sperm banks directly reflected the principles and personal politics of the founders. Each of these philosophical positions is in some way a belief in eugenics—the promotion of the reproduction of certain groups of people over others to varying degrees. These beliefs permeate the industry at a variety of levels, including how donors and clients are screened and selected, the sexual orientation of donors and recipients, how semen is perceived, and the continuum of identity release and concealment.

These different sperm banks appeal to different types of men to become donors, with different motivations, levels of desire for compensation, and prospects for future contact with the intended mothers or the children born from their sperm. Some men become known donors for women they know and do not receive financial compensation at all. Some sperm bank donors—for example, at RGC—also received no compensation and were recruited to "improve the human gene pool" because they were perceived by the repository to be "exceptional men." RGC donors were to forever remain anonymous. RFHS only provided a modest amount of reimbursement for "time and trouble," and donors who provided there were more motivated by a desire to have some connection with the child born from their sperm. RFHS provided mothers with their donor's contact information when their child was three months old. TSBC donors could either agree to have their identity released to the child when he or she turned eighteen or remain anonymous. Men's decisions to provide sperm at one sperm bank over another, or to provide for someone known by the donor rather than a sperm bank, are directly connected to their own reasons for becoming a donor in the first place.

The founding principles that guided each of the banks resulted in different reproductive goals. These sites are not just places where reproductive services are provided; they are all guiding reproduction—using technology—according to the personal convictions of their founders. The policies at these practices represent conflicting notions of who is fit to be a genetic parent (donor) and who is fit to have and raise children (recipient). These agendas are both personal and political.

3 · SEMEN TO GO
Choosing Conception Alternatively

I never know what to call it, this whole new world, the "semen to go"
language. I go, "I need a to-go order," and they don't seem to quite have my
sense of humor.   —Carolyn

One's own body is in the world just as the heart is in the organism.
                                          —Maurice Merleau-Ponty (1944, 245)

     The quest for parenthood is ordinary, irrespective of marital status or
sexual orientation. But with the choice to have a child through donor insemination,
maternity is transformed into something extraordinary. The process of getting
semen to go, as if one were ordering a hamburger through a fast-food drive-up
window, seems a highly unusual route to parenthood, but the act is integrated
into the mundane tasks of everyday life. Semen samples, nestled in liquid
nitrogen tanks and six-pack coolers, are driven around town in the back seats of
women's cars, sharing the space with groceries and dry cleaning. Seeking motherhood through donor insemination leads to a heightened awareness of the body,
redefines the mundane, and can alter one's sense of self and how one experiences
the world.
     Several themes emerged from my interviews with women pursuing mother-
hood, some with female partners and some on their own. Notions of aging, relationships, biological and social kinship, and the meaning of fatherhood, as well
as fears of infertility, all came up in our conversations. Women seeking motherhood on their own confront somewhat different issues from women who seek to
build families with their female partners—the latter of whom in many ways reflect
the same motivations for parenthood as straight couples do—but there are over-
lapping experiences these women share.
     Embarking on the decision to have a child through donor insemination opens
a clinical world that fuses both the familiar and the alien, as Rebecca relayed in
her story about picking up sperm to go:

I remember how it used to be when I would go there for a "pickup." I'll never forget how the elevator button feels; it's a texture in your mind. It's going to be there forever. . . . Up the elevator, ring the bell, "I'm here for a pickup." Sit in that little room. . . . Then I'd get this tank, and put it in the back seat of my car. My car is not equipped [for] carrying nitrogen tanks and things, and it [the tank] would tip over and I'd think, "Oh my God, it's tipped over. What are happening to the little sperm getting splashed around in the tank?" And sometimes I would actually forget it was in the back of my car and I'd be driving all around Berkeley with this tank full of sperm. I once had to go through hypnotherapy to help lessen my anxiety about sperm pickup.

Getting semen to go transforms one's perceptions of self and body. To borrow from Maurice Merleau-Ponty (1944), the phenomenological sensations of something as commonplace as the touch of an elevator button take on new significance. The bodily sensations can remain even years later.

CHOOSING MOTHERHOOD ALTERNATIVELY

Single Mothers by Choice

I first met Rebecca at her cozy Berkeley cottage on a cool February afternoon in 1997. She opened her door and welcomed me into her home, where I noticed the immaculate shine of her hardwood floors; a plush, white living-room sofa with an afghan throw nestled beneath the sizable front window; and the aroma of a steaming vegetable omelet accompanied by a cup of hot, black coffee. Rebecca, forty and a psychologist, had arrived home from a long day of appointments with her clients and quickly pulled together dinner before my anticipated arrival. Between bites of her omelet, she told me about her declining fertility: "You know, I made the decision to do this alone, and I'm like, 'OK, I'm never going to have a lover again.' I thought that early on. It's been kind of scary—all the aspects of doing this alone—it's scary to think that, physically you won't be attractive to people, and it's kind of fucking scary to be forty anyway. And, being single, forty, and trying to get pregnant and having no children, and forty and being single. I feel like my head is going to explode."

Rebecca not only felt overwhelmed by having just turned forty but also felt like a failure because she had not been able to find a suitable husband to have a child with. She said, "I did everything right: went to college, went to graduate school, got a good job, bought a house, and have been responsible. Everything I've set out to do, I've accomplished—except this one thing, finding a stable relationship to bring a child into. That one thing makes me feel like I've failed as a woman. My parents never prepared me for this!"

Rebecca was part of a growing trend of single women choosing motherhood without a male partner. One of the main factors that influences women's decisions to pursue motherhood—especially single, straight women—is aging. Research on family formation in Spain demonstrates that, as in the United States, people are waiting longer to have children, economic constraints play into delayed child-bearing, and aging is a major factor in people's decisions to have children when they do (Konvalinka 2013). For heterosexual single mothers by choice, in both Spain and the United States, the decision to have a child alone is usually perceived as a last resort in the face of one's waning reproductive years (Miller 1992; Hertz, Rivas, and Jociles 2016). As Gay Becker's extensive research on infertility and the life course demonstrates, for women who struggle to conceive, or who are unsuc-cessful, it feels like a complete disruption of life course (Becker 1990, 1994, 2000; Friese, Becker and Nachtigall 2006). For single, heterosexual women who want a partner or husband and have not found one, and who want a child and have not been able to have one, the feelings of failure are extreme and are accompanied by a profound sense of having no control over one's life and vision for the future.

Throughout my interviews with single women, I heard repeated concerns about their "eggs getting old," and fears they would not be able to reproduce if they waited much longer. Almost every single woman I interviewed cited her age as a decid-ing factor in seeking motherhood on her own when she did. Most women saw thirty-five as a milestone for making the decision to have a child through donor insemination, and interview participants repeatedly cited medical research that shows women over thirty-five have significantly decreased fertility. This aware-ness of medical research on infertility after thirty-five came up over and over again, to the point that it was incorporated into women's perceptions of themselves, their bodies, and their notions of aging.

As women reached their late thirties or early forties, the sense of urgency, and feelings of hopelessness surrounding their bodies' ability to conceive, increased. Many women resented these "medical facts" and the recurrent messages from medical practitioners that "time was running out." As Stanley Brandes (1987) notes, women increasingly view forty as a time of midlife crisis, which is rooted in cultural perceptions of aging. However, women in my study were concerned with the "biological facts" of decreased fertility that comes with increasing age. This was compounded by the perception that a loss of sexual attractiveness accom-panied declining fertility due to aging.

In 1981 Jane Mattes launched a support group known as Single Mothers by Choice. The group quickly became a national, then international, organization, with thousands of women considering or embarking on motherhood on their own. The emergence of this group was part of a larger trend in a number of West-ern countries in which the stigma of unmarried mothers began to decline—albeit slowly. By 1991, single motherhood by choice was establishing a presence on main-stream television with the character Murphy Brown. Despite the conservative political environment and Dan Quayle's Murphy Brown speech (quoted in chap-ter 1), many of the single women I spoke with who were trying to conceive through donor insemination mentioned the Murphy Brown character as a model for successful (straight) single motherhood.

For most heterosexual women, the decision to move forward with using a sperm donor was not their first choice. Most single, straight women who decided to become a parent through sperm donation—or even through more informal channels such as conceiving as a result of a one-night stand—expressed a desire to become a mother "the right way." Many went through a mourning process before deciding to choose motherhood alone. Many feared their reproductive time was running out and still held out hope that the right man would come along, perhaps after they had their child. Carolyn described her feelings about marriage and single motherhood: "I figured out around thirty that if I didn't find anybody I wanted to marry—by about thirty-five or thirty-four is the number I had put in my mind—I would look into a way to have kids on my own and have a family on my own because that was important whether or not I was married. I figured I could get married anytime but at least that would be the point for my body that I would need to start deciding if I was going to have kids myself."

For Carolyn, the ability to have children was limited by time, but finding someone to marry was not. For her, having a husband was not a necessary requirement for having a child, even if it was preferable. As Carolyn approached forty, the sense of urgency to conceive a child increased dramatically. Rebecca experienced this urgency as an identity crisis. Josie echoes this feeling: "When I was thirty-eight I woke up on my birthday and all of the sudden I was obsessed with having a baby. All I could think about was baby, baby, baby, baby, baby. It was some kind of identity crisis, but I just couldn't shake it."

Perceptions of aging are connected to popular perceptions of the limitations of the biological, fertile, female body, and they are a major factor in determining when women decide to attempt pregnancy. These notions of aging and fertility are strongly connected to women's perceptions of themselves as feminine and sexually attractive, especially for heterosexual women or those who identified as more on the feminine side of the gender spectrum. Even though sexuality and reproduction are separated through technology, some women still perceived them as conflated in their sense of self.

The Lesbian Baby Boom

The mid-1980s witnessed another emerging trend pushing the traditional boundaries of family—the so-called lesbian baby boom. This was especially true in the San Francisco Bay Area. For lesbian couples, aging did factor into the decision of when to start trying to conceive, but this was not perceived as connected to the inability to find an adequate partner. However, getting access to sperm—especially before sperm banks opened their doors to single women and lesbian couples—required some consideration. Karleen Pendleton Jiménez, in her personal memoir, *How to Get a Girl Pregnant*, asks, "How do I get sperm when I look like a dude and I'm older and fatter than when I used to pick up guys as a teenager?" (2011, 5). Like many women, she struggled with whether to choose a known donor or a sperm bank donor on her path to parenthood, but she also grappled with her own Chicana, butch, lesbian identity as she observed and attempted to participate in the heterosexual mate-attraction process. Jiménez grappled with whether to use a known donor or a sperm bank donor and came to the conclusion that, while a sperm bank donor may protect the boundaries of her lesbian nuclear family, she actually wanted to know the donor was not "creepy" and wanted an actual friendship with him—both for her own sake and for the sake of her future child.

Pepper (thirty-eight) and Karen (thirty-nine) had been friends for many years before becoming involved romantically. When they first met, Karen was married to a man but was having problems in her marriage. Pepper was out as a lesbian and had just gone through a breakup, and Karen was trying to fix her up with another lesbian friend of hers at work, where she was a software developer. As she was describing Pepper to her other friend, trying to set them up on a date, suddenly Karen realized she had feelings for Pepper. As Karen explained, "It was a shock to me. And it wasn't that I was looking for a woman. I was looking for Pepper. I didn't define myself when I first came out as a lesbian. It's just that as I was describing her and all her wonderful qualities I realized I was in love with her."

Karen divorced her husband. After several years together, Karen and Pepper decided it was time to have a child, and Karen wanted to be the one to carry. They started exploring resources in the Bay Area for LGBT family building, like The Alternative Family Project and MAIA Midwifery, where they attended a number of classes on their family-building options. After some consideration, they decided they were more comfortable using a sperm bank donor than a known donor because they wanted to make sure that they would be the only parents, that they would not have to incorporate a donor into their family, and that Pepper's role as the nonbiological mother would be protected. They eventually signed up at a number of sperm banks in search of the right donor, preferably someone with Italian heritage, like Pepper. Their donor was based out of a sperm bank in Los Angeles, so they had the semen samples shipped.

PEPPER: The sperm bank FedExed the sperm to me at my work. So the tank would show up at my work every month and the receptionist kept asking me what was in it. We didn't tell anyone we were trying. Finally she asked, "Is it helium?" And I said yes, because I didn't think it was any of her business.

Then I'd meet Karen for dinner before going home and we'd have this FedEx box with us at the dinner table. And people would give us these weird looks. I just wanted to tell everyone, "It's semen, OK?" So we'd be sitting there, having a romantic dinner, with our glasses of wine and our tank of sperm.

KAREN: I wanted to feel like Pepper got me pregnant. So we'd have our typical Friday night date night, go home and light some candles and put on some music, and then Pepper would do the insemination. It took a couple years to get pregnant, and we were about to give up; I was becoming a basket case. Finally, the doctor put me on Clomid and we just had our baby daughter four months ago.

For Pepper and Karen, getting sperm from a sperm bank helped preserve the nuclear family model that was important to them. Unlike people who use known sperm donors, those who use sperm banks have more legal and social protection over their relationship to their child and the boundaries of their family. Taking the sperm on a date and creating a romantic setting for insemination, rather than a clinical one, made for a more relaxed environment in which to conceive and ensured both that Pepper had an active role in their conception and that their child was created and born out of their love for each other.

Sperm banks offer clients access to a large selection of donors. Women can peruse donor profiles to find men who have the traits they are looking for, including physical traits like hair and eye color and other traits such as education and hobbies. Some sperm banks offer donors willing to have their identity released when the offspring reaches eighteen, so they have the option of connecting in the future. At one sperm bank where I conducted interviews with staff, sperm from "identity release" donors cost more per vial than sperm from donors who wished to remain forever anonymous. Since more women wanted to have options available for their potential offspring, identity-release sperm was in higher demand. Bonnie told me why using an open-identity donor was important to her and her partner, Sharon: "My father died when I was four, and I'm an only child, so it was just my mother and me when I was growing up. So for me, having a donor who the kid can know when they grow up, that's an important issue. Lots of people give sperm and aren't willing to be known. But growing up, people always asked me, 'What does your father do?' And I couldn't answer. I want our kid to be able to find out when they grow up so they don't always wonder."

Some women chose known donors, a friend or a person they met through social networks or possibly by advertising online. Occasionally, known donors and recipients enter into co-parenting arrangements, whereby the donor is involved in the child's life to varying degrees. Usually, women and men who enter into agreements have an attorney draw up contracts that clearly delineate each parent's rights and responsibilities in regard to the child. Some women advertised for donors through gay or lesbian presses, on website forums, or on Craigslist and made private arrangements to buy sperm directly, but among the women I spoke to, these were comparatively few.

Kira, twenty-eight, refers to herself as a "bisexual dyke." She used a friend as a known donor. When the HIV/AIDS crisis struck, it affected her personally, as well as a number of her friends, and changed how many lesbians chose donors. She said,

> It's not like lesbian women haven't been getting pregnant for ages. But they used to use known donors, or go-betweens if they wanted an unknown donor in order to get semen. And then came along HIV and messed that up for everybody. It really hit me personally. My best friend wanted to be a known donor. We negotiated everything and we did the insemination. And then he tested positive for HIV, so he couldn't have any more kids after that. It was really scary! Then I had to get an HIV test because we didn't know if he was positive before or after I conceived. I went through my pregnancy not knowing. Not only was it terrifying, but it changed our whole relationship. At first, I planned on just being a single parent. But after we found out his status, we renegotiated things so he could be a co-parent, because this was the only child he would ever have.

In the 1980s and 1990s, the HIV/AIDS crisis sent shockwaves through the LGBTQ community. Not only were people dying in droves, but homosexual men were suddenly cast in a high-risk category as potential transmitters of disease. Paul Farmer's (1992) work on HIV, *Aids and Accusation,* addresses the stigma facing high-risk groups—homosexuals, hemophiliacs, Haitians, and heroin addicts—and how the geography of blame actually exacerbated the public health threat of HIV. Sarah Franklin (1993) further demonstrates how the HIV/AIDS crisis, combined with assisted reproductive technologies, further reinforced homophobia and stigma against LGBTQ communities. Notions of homosexuality and risk were exemplified by Food and Drug Administration guidelines barring men who had sex with men from being sperm donors at sperm banks. Many women in the LGBTQ community, though, wanted to use known gay sperm donors. And many gay men wanted to be known sperm donors, so they could have some role in a child's life.

Some lesbian women seeking motherhood through sperm donation felt the risk of using a gay man as a known donor to be too great and turned to sperm banks instead, where semen samples were quarantined for six months and the donors were tested and retested for HIV. For other women, it was more important to have a gay man as a known donor so the child would have a connection to him, and they minimized the risk by having their donor get tested and retested six months later, with no sexual activity in between, or choosing someone who was not sexually active.

Becky (forty-one) and Janine (thirty-seven) had been trying to conceive for a year; Becky started trying when she was thirty-three on her own and in other relationships that subsequently broke up. Janine already had a son when she and Becky met. I asked Becky how she and her partner went about choosing a donor. She explained,

We'd advertised in one of the gay/lesbian newspapers. And at that time we got quite a lot of guys, and we chose him because he was gay, but he had been celibate for many, many years, like ten years. He had had many HIV tests, which were negative. So he seemed medically safe and I preferred the idea of a gay donor as opposed to a straight donor. . . . I mean, it's much harder for a gay man to come along years later and say she's a lesbian so she shouldn't be raising my child. I find it very hard to trust that a straight man might not do that at some point. I felt really confident that he wanted to have a child. He didn't want to be overly involved. It was the right setup, it seemed. I felt that he wanted just the right amount of involvement. It felt right that he be a known donor. I mean, we had a written agreement and it was clear I was going to be the parent.

Women who used known donors usually relied on contracts and agreements to nullify the donor's parental rights, absolve him of any financial responsibilities, and define the amount of contact he would have with the child. Most articulated that the mothers were the sole parents, with full legal, financial, and social responsibility for caring for their child. At the time, the nonbiological mother would have to go through a lengthy and costly second-parent adoption process in order to have her parental rights recognized, but this option was not available in every county or every state. For some couples, using a known donor was seen as a possible threat to the nonbiological co-mother and her relationship to her child, with some nonbiological mothers feeling jealous of the donor, the biological mother, or both (Pelka 2009). At a time when women who came out as lesbian during a divorce were losing custody of their children (Lewin 1993), it was particularly important to take whatever steps were necessary to protect their donor-conceived families legally. A man who wanted to be more actively involved, and have a role more like that of a father, most likely would not be chosen to be a donor.

By choosing a sperm bank donor instead of a known donor, some lesbian co-parents form families that parallel heterosexual nuclear families. By not having a donor involved, the family consists of two parents, their donor-conceived children, and, to varying degrees, their respective extended families. Couples with known donors, however, may incorporate their donor on a spectrum of involvement in the child's life, from minimal contact to regular contact, and may also include donor-extended kinship into their families (Sullivan 2004).

CONSTRUCTING KINSHIP

It is only in the past twenty-five years that anthropologists have paid attention to how women define their own families. Carol Stack's (1974) *All Our Kin* emphasizes the significance of social relations, more so than biological relatedness, in the definition of family in a poor black community. This work demonstrates how children's kinship is determined by the women who raised them. Here, it is the matrilineal ties that are considered significant, and Stack's informants considered the man who helped raise them to be more significant than the man who is their biological father. As one of her informants told her, "Starting down the street from here, take my father, he ain't my daddy, he's no father to me. I ain't got but one daddy and that's Jason. The one who raised me" (45). Here, Stack notes how the categories of "father" (the biological relationship) and "daddy" (the social relationship) have different meanings. Many of the women in my research also had fathers who did not raise them, asserted that biology does not make a dad, and drew on the distinction between biological and social fatherhood in forming their decision to use a sperm donor to have a child.

In her analysis of assisted reproductive technologies and kinship in England, Marilyn Strathern writes, "If till now kinship has been a symbol for everything that cannot be changed about social affairs, if biology has been a symbol for the given parameters of human existence, what will it mean for the way we construe any of our relationships with one another to think of parenting as the implementing of an option and genetic make-up as an outcome of cultural preference?" (1992b, 34). Kinship has been dramatically altered by the uses of reproductive technologies, which have restructured biological and social kin ties. Reproductive technologies have led to different and more complex ways of identifying and thinking about the family, including the separation of biological and social parenthood, and parenting involves an active decision to parent a child and is not a biological given.

The use of reproductive technologies specifically challenges traditional models of kinship and magnifies the myriad possibilities for kinship beyond biology. The model of the family as a heterosexual, married couple and their offspring is also challenged. Much of the literature in lesbian and gay studies has also challenged the significance of biological kin ties, noting that, in the words of Kath Weston ([1991] 1997), families are "the families we choose." Although much of this work has focused on the alienation LGBTQ people experience when coming out to their families of origin, which thereby creates the need to define their own social kin networks, it points to the significance of alternative kinship systems.

Weston ([1991] 1997) demonstrates the cultural relativity of kinship and gender and sexual identity. Important here is the flexibility in defining kin within LGBTQ communities, in which social kin is often prioritized over biological kin. Her work points to different ways in which the family is constructed. Donor insemination adds another twist to fluctuating definitions of kinship and procreation—and "challenges conventional understanding of biological offspring" (Weston [1991] 1997, 169). For example, one of my informants had a child with her female partner using a known donor. When the child was delivered, the partner's name was put on the birth certificate where the father's name would normally go. Although this does not legally identify the partner as a parent, this couple considered the act to be symbolically and politically significant. The partner who did not deliver the child was later able to legally adopt and is now a legal mother. The biological father, or donor, visits the child often and is considered to have "uncle" status. This exemplifies how social kin are redefined—the child has both a biosocial mother and a social mother—but also how biological relationships are redefined—the child has an uncle in lieu of a father.

Among the women in my study, the definition of family is fluid and a biological father's involvement in a child's life is not perceived as necessary to the development of a healthy child. These are not new arguments. Whether through divorce, "accidental pregnancies," or donor insemination, women create and sustain families on their own, without men. Among many women deciding to parent alone, or with a female partner, there is the notion that a child born to a loving mother will not be disadvantaged by a father's absence.

I met Anna and Joanne at their upstairs Victorian flat, nestled in San Francisco's Noe Valley neighborhood. Anna explained how they wrestled with the decision of whether to pursue using a known donor, with whom a future child could have contact, or an anonymous donor. Anna did not feel a father figure's presence was necessary for a child to be well adjusted, as long as there was a wider network of social and familial support:

> I think that one of the processes I had to go through when arriving at this decision to have a child without a "father" being present is [to realize that] Joanne grew up without her father, but has turned out beautifully, I think. And because she has these other people in her life, like her grandparents, she has grown up with a lot of support. I grew up with my father, and I think all my siblings and I can certainly say that we're worse for wear of having our father there. So, in my mind . . . I don't see that a father is absolutely a necessary person to have in raising a child to a healthy, balanced point. I think it would be nice for the child to simply have that option to know the person, but I don't think that person needs to be there in order for the child to turn out OK.

Research supports the notion that donor-conceived children raised in single and same-sex households grow up well adjusted (Scheib and Hastings 2012) and that most want access to information or connection to their donors (Scheib, Riordan, and Rubin 2005; Scheib, Ruby, and Benward 2017). Many women having children without male partners choose to use an identity release or a known donor so their child can have access to the donor's information should he or she want it. Most women who opt for known donors over sperm bank donors hope any child conceived will have some sort of relationship with the donor, but usually not one where the donor assumes the role of father.

Joanne and Anna agreed they wanted to use a known donor so their child had the option of knowing who the donor is, but they wanted his relationship with the child to be limited and controlled by a legal contract. For women using known donors, there is always the consideration of how much contact there will be between the donor and the child. Thus, recognition of paternity and donor involvement are negotiated between the contracting parties, but laws differ from state to state and contracts may not be legally binding in all states.

Another decision lesbian couples face is determining which partner will attempt to conceive. For some couples, there is clearly one woman who wants to experience pregnancy and one who does not. Other couples may take turns, with one woman attempting to conceive their first child, and the other their second, often both using the same donor so that the donor-conceived children can be half siblings biologically. For others, the decision regarding who is going to try to conceive is more a medical one—for example, if one partner is older and less likely to be able to conceive or has known fertility issues. And some couples decide to retrieve eggs from one partner to be carried by the other partner, so that they both have a biological attachment to the child.

The relationship between donor and child is negotiated and controlled by the women who seek pregnancy. Some women feel comfortable with co-parenting arrangements in which the donor has certain rights and responsibilities in relation to the offspring. Other women contract to have complete parental autonomy in regard to the child and offer the donor a limited relationship to the child; likewise, the donor has limited responsibilities in regard to care for the child and is not responsible for payment of child support.

Women who used Rainbow Flag Health Services were required to make contact with the donor when the child turned three months old. But they were able to determine how much contact to have with the donor once he became known. Women who used open-identity donors offered their child the option to meet their donor when the child turned eighteen years old, but it was not possible for the child to have a relationship with the donor before reaching adulthood. Some women choose anonymous, or non-identity-release, donors who have no involvement in their child's life and, presumably, no potential for future contact. The relationship between a child and biological father (donor) is determined by the mother. The treatment of donor identities, then, is negotiated by the inseminating mother or couple and is dependent on women's interpretation—and experience—of the significance of fatherhood in children's lives. It is important to note, however, that even though people did not realize it at the time, donor anonymity could not be guaranteed indefinitely. By 2000, Wendy Kramer and her donor-conceived son, Ryan, founded the Donor Sibling Registry. This registry enables children conceived with the same donor to be in contact with one another, as well as with donor-conceived children and their donors. More recently, both donors and donor-conceived children have been using direct-to-consumer DNA test kits, ancestry websites, and social networking and registry sites like donor children.com to find one another. Regardless of the original intentions of the mother or mothers, as their children matured, many took the quest for connection with biological kin into their own hands.

For many of the single women I interviewed, the notion prevailed that biological fathers are not necessarily important, that fatherhood is an unstable, fluctuating category that is socially—rather than biologically—situated. Many either were raised by their mothers or, if there was a father figure in the picture, felt more of an attachment to their stepfather than to their biological father. Others had a biological father who lived elsewhere and was not involved in their lives. And some had fathers who were simply inaccessible. Men, for a number of these women, were not necessary for creating a family and were, in fact, viewed as largely replaceable.

Sandy was a white, thirty-eight-year-old mother of three, and graduate student at Berkeley. She saw a connection between her experiences with her own biological father and her decision to have her third child through donor insemination:

> Growing up there was a funny kind of system of kinship where male kin were always fluctuating. There were always new fathers and it was very unstable in that way. My mother was divorced—my father left her for another woman when I was three or four and I've never seen him or heard from him since. So she married my stepfather, and he really has been my father, and we're pretty close too. I've thought a lot about whether or not to look my biological father up and I've made the decision not to because, to me, a father is a person who is responsible and plays that role, and *he* never sent a birthday card, *he* never made any contact.
>
> But it was really this idea that he could just leave one family and start another, and that made me feel that men were replaceable. So I think what I based my decision on was that I didn't see him as my father beyond a certain point. And I guess that's where I really started to question the whole business of what is a genetic father and why do we give it so much meaning, because here's somebody who absolutely was not involved in my life at all, yet people always say, well, where's your *real* father?

Having been raised in a blended family seems to help women rebel against limits on their reproductive options. For example, Sandy discussed how her upbringing caused her to see fatherhood as more socially than biologically based. This perspective also aided her in making the decision to choose to have her third child through donor insemination.

At the time of our interview, Sandy was seven months pregnant by a donor from a sperm bank, and she was a graduate student at the University of California, Berkeley. Sandy is one of seven children. She became pregnant at the age of sixteen, with her first daughter, Trisha, "to get out of the house because it was an unbearable situation. My stepdad would sometimes drink and get pretty violent."

She never considered her first daughter's father as someone she would marry, but she has "had a good relationship with him over the years" and describes him as a friend. When she was twenty-two, she got pregnant and married the father of her second daughter, Maggie.

"When he found out I was pregnant, though, he was sort of the 'classic ass' about it: He said, 'How do I know it's mine?' . . . He tried to contest paternity. Of course, he lost. I made the decision to have her realizing I was probably going to be on my own. . . . He wouldn't even acknowledge her." Sandy told me what the breakup of her marriage meant to her.

> I wanted to be married and have a baby and do it right. . . . It was very traumatic for me because I really wanted the marriage to work and he didn't. I felt my daughter deserved to have a father . . . and when I was about seven months pregnant he had an affair. And then he basically said, "See ya."
>
> It was really a terrible time. At that point I decided I'm going to raise my two girls. Trisha's father was very funny. He always considered Maggie to be his daughter too. If he came to take Trisha out he took Maggie out too. And again, it's that recurring theme for me in my life that parenthood is social. The difference in my life has been that the people who have consistently been there have not been biological relatives. You make your own family.

Sandy then told me how she decided to have a child through donor insemination. Since she turned thirty-five, she wanted to have another baby and thought about it a lot. She was twenty-three when her daughter Maggie was born, and she thought she would eventually meet someone but did not.

> So, for a couple of years I would say jokingly, "Well, I think I'll just go to the sperm bank," as sort of this ridiculous joke that, of course, I would never do. And then I started talking to people and reading and, you know how when something is in the back of your mind you start noticing, so I would notice that in the paper there were articles on debating the ethical issues. Then I met some people who became good friends, a lesbian couple, who live in Albany and have two girls that are twelve and fourteen who were conceived by artificial insemination. They were some of the first people at the California Sperm Bank. They're just a really good couple and really good parents. I really respected the way they said, "We wanted to build a family and to hell with the social controls that exist to make it so hard." I think each of them had had one of the children and used the same donor.
>
> When I talk with other single moms over age thirty-five—a certain recognition Mr. Prince Charming wasn't coming by on the horse anytime soon and if I held my breath too much longer my options would be really limited. My kids were getting older and I realized how much I enjoyed being a parent and how cheated I felt because my life was so in crisis when I had them. It was at that point,

right when I hit thirty-five, that I thought maybe it's too late now and maybe there's not going to be the right person. Then I got pregnant accidentally and had a miscarriage. I was so devastated and I felt an incredible sense of panic about time running out. I felt this real urgency and had this big question mark about maybe I'm just too old. Maybe I miscarried because the eggs have gone bad. They're just too old.

So I went to the sperm bank. It was an interesting experience because on the one hand I've got this person explaining the procedures and showing me how it works and everything and I'm listening as a client, and on the other hand I'm listening from a very critical standpoint going, "What is this all about?" and about the ethics of it all. I guess the thing that surprised me the most is how quickly all of the ethical issues, and things that have actually come out recently for me again, like what do you tell the child and all that, totally faded into the background because of the quest to get pregnant. It becomes this overriding thing. Financially it was a strain because it was $250 just to go through the orientation and then 110 bucks a pop and you wanted to use at least two samples each month. Of course, what starts happening, and I talked to many other people who had this experience, is you start buying three and four because you think you'll just optimize my chances. I'll inseminate twice a day for three days and that's six. This is one of the advantages I think of having a partner—the sperm is free.

I feel a certain doubt about meeting someone because I think, right now, my life is pretty full and it's not a number one priority—whereas in my twenties it was. I mean, that would be wonderful. I'd love to have a partner but only a partner who shared my interests and loved my kids and the chances of finding that, especially in the society we live in, seems to me to be very small. . . . Plus, I have three kids by three different fathers: one I divorced and one I wasn't married to and one I went to the sperm bank, and I'm in my late thirties. So on the list of marriageable qualities, I don't think I'm high on anyone's list. And I'm not willing to do what it seems to me so many women do—make sacrifices to be in a relationship. I don't want it that bad. Not at any cost. I've seen what bad parents can do to kids and it really scares me.

For many straight, single women, the decision to have a child through donor insemination is thoroughly entangled with fears of aging, not wanting to wait for a relationship to have a child and thereby possibly sacrificing their ability to conceive, and also not wanting to make the sacrifice of being in a bad relationship. Furthermore, the instability of male kin in one's family history provides many women with a model for thinking about the family that renders the paternal involvement in child-rearing insignificant, problematic, or, at worst (as in the following case), disastrous.

Carolyn was a thirty-five-year-old single, heterosexual woman of European ancestry with two siblings who was raised by a single mother. She had been undergoing donor insemination for six months but had not yet conceived. She attributed her ability to make the decision to have a child on her own to her upbringing in a single-parent household, as well as her parents' poor role modeling in marital relationships: "I think that we didn't have any models for good relationships. Mom and Dad were awful and then my dad married another woman and that was awful. . . . For me, the decision to go it alone is measured on 'Can you support yourself'? Then it's like 'OK, you can add these other layers.'"

For Carolyn and many others, the decision to have a child on one's own is directly connected to having emerged from a family with "failed kinship"—where the "father" was either absent (under a variety of circumstances) or "fluctuating." However, this failure at kinship—with both fathers and husbands or lovers—has a positive side: it also gives women the perspective that it is possible for them to parent on their own, and that a bad relationship is too much of a sacrifice. Although some women express sorrow at not having men in their lives, there is also a sense of confidence that they can raise a child alone and provide him or her with a healthy, stable environment. Economic independence also factors into the decision.

Despite being raised in a social environment in which single parenthood is acceptable, these same women express a conflicting wish to have "the ideal"—the nuclear family with the husband, wife, two kids, and so on. Like Sandy, many women express the fact that, given their age and other circumstances, they do not think "Prince Charming" will be arriving anytime soon. There is often a sense of loss or failure at relationships, as well as the belief that a woman has to compromise too much to find a reasonable partner. Age, then, is a primary factor in women's decisions to choose single motherhood—the notion that one's fertility is a limited resource. Yet, for women, the decision to go through the process of donor insemination alone is, to some degree, a statement that one is, at least temporarily, giving up on marriage. Indeed, several straight women, like Rebecca, explained to me how they had become involved in relationships that they normally would have avoided simply because the man expressed the desire to have a baby with them:

> When I first started inseminating I was seeing this guy and I told him what I was going to do. And he was like "Oh, great, I want to join you; I want to have a baby with you; I want to be the father; I want to be the sperm donor or anything else you'll give me." I was with him for a few months. . . . He turned out to be a really complicated person, and he wasn't really who I thought he was . . . and I had this feeling that I really opened myself up to this situation, and I had been with someone I would never have usually considered just because he wanted to have a child with me. I haven't really been involved with anyone since.

Women undergoing donor insemination perceive the experience differently according to relationship status and sexual orientation. For one bisexual woman,

Deena (twenty-six), having a partner—male or female—was completely irrelevant to her quest to have a child:

> I always wanted to have a child when I was young, like in my twenties, like my mom.
> She's in her fifties now and her kids are gone and she's off traveling around the world
> and enjoying her life. And I'm bisexual, so I never had that thing about waiting for
> the right guy—and I can't imagine trusting anyone enough to have a child with—
> so I didn't see any reason to wait. So I was turning twenty-six and as a birthday
> gift to myself I went to the sperm bank and got started. I figured, "What? I'm not
> going to have kids because I don't have a lover?" That's so stupid! I want to have
> kids. I want to be a parent now.

But most single women in my study, regardless of sexual orientation, tended
to view the decision to have a child alone as coming to terms with relationship
failure, as Carolyn explained: "Deciding to go through this alone is like saying no
one would want me. It's giving up on the whole Prince Charming and white picket
fence idea. Well, maybe not the white picket fence—I can buy that if I want—
but this is certainly not the way I always thought about having kids."

This notion of failure at relationships pervaded my interviews with single
women of all sexual orientations. For most of these women, there was the fairy-
tale notion they grew up with—they would fall in love, get married, have children,
and have the perfect conventional family—even though many of these women
grew up in homes where the father had left, was an alcoholic, was abusive, or was
inaccessible. Many of these women reported feeling betrayed because social expectations for family did not match their experiences with family relations, for
themselves or their children.

For many women, it would be preferable, if not always possible, to have a partner rather than parent alone. For example, Monica, a thirty-five-year-old single,
bisexual woman said, "Doing this [insemination] alone has been really hard.
I would much rather have a partner through all of this. It doesn't matter to me if
it's a woman or a man, just someone who can share the ups and downs, someone
who will love this child as much as I do."

CREATING FAMILIES ALTERNATIVELY

Single women and lesbian couples have different considerations when deciding
to have children. For many single women, the decision to have a child on one's
own is made due to the lack of an adequate partner. Many women said they would
rather have a child with a partner but found themselves no longer willing to wait
for the right partner to come along, especially when facing concerns around aging
and declining fertility.

Unlike single women, lesbian couples I spoke to saw donor insemination as a normal part of the process of starting a family. For them, like most heterosexual couples, having a child was viewed as a normal outgrowth of their relationship and their commitment to one another—even if the method of conception was not conventional by society's standards. As one woman told me, "We [lesbians] have more sense of control over trying to get pregnant than heterosexual women do because, for us, donor insemination is a normal process." Ellen Lewin echoed this in a presentation at the American Anthropological Association meetings in Philadelphia, in 1998: "For lesbians, donor insemination is a perfectly natural method of conceiving a child—how else would a lesbian get pregnant?" The motivations for lesbian couples to have children, then, are not that different from heterosexual couples', but they may require technological assistance in order to become parents.

In the 1990s, though, lesbian couples faced numerous challenges to having their families legally and socially recognized. Many also faced obstacles to getting insemination treatment—especially if they experienced difficulties conceiving. For heterosexual, married couples, any offspring conceived during that union are considered legally to be the offspring of the husband, even if he is not the biological parent. Thus the husband, the presumed father of the child, has a legally protected relationship in case of divorce or the death of the spouse.

For the nonbiological lesbian mother in the 1990s, however, her status as co-parent of the child was not recognized, in part because the relationship was not legally recognized. If the couple separated, the biological mother would be considered the sole legal parent and the nonbiological mother had no rights or responsibilities whatsoever—regardless of whether she and her partner entered into the pregnancy together. For example, in one California case, *Crandall v. Wagner*, the nonbiological mother was denied visitation rights to a child she and her partner had conceived together through donor insemination and they had raised together for over five years.[1] The court did recognize that Crandall, the nonbiological mother, had been a de facto parent, but she had not legally adopted the child and thus was found to have no claims to visitation rights.

In California, up until 2005, all custody cases involving lesbian mothers who were not biological or adoptive mothers had been lost. The first California child custody case to grant custody and visitation was *K.M. v. E.G.*[2] In this case, K. M. had donated eggs to her partner, E. G., so that her partner could carry the pregnancy and K. M. would be the biological parent. This is an approach that is often used in lesbian relationships so that both partners have a biological or genetic link to the child. Unfortunately, the fertility clinic required that K. M. act as a typical "egg donor" and relinquish any parental rights. The couple conceived twins, carried by E. G. A few years later, the couple separated, and E. G. claimed she was the only legal mother of the twins, denying her partner parental rights. The California Supreme Court decided that the contract through the fertility center was null and void, that the couple entered into the conception with the intent to parent together, and therefore that K. M. should be awarded rights to custody and visitation.

As in custody disputes, if the biological mother in a same-sex couple died, the nonbiological mother had no rights to the child, who could then be placed with blood relatives of the biological mother. For many lesbian couples, the challenges of having their family recognized—along with the fear that a known donor could challenge their rights as parents and claim custody—led to feelings of vulnerability.

The inherent challenges of co-parenting as lesbian mothers informed many women's decisions to use a sperm bank donor. Judy and Kim first thought about using a friend as a known donor but then decided on a sperm bank donor for this reason. Judy explained their decision: "We briefly discussed getting it from this friend of ours, but we dismissed that almost right away, because we didn't want any kind of complication. You don't want a known donor coming along and claiming paternity and all that stuff, even if there's a contract. So we went to the sperm bank, they gave us this listing and it felt like the safest way to start a family— especially since Kim is going to have to go through the second-parent adoptions, we just didn't want any complications."

At the time, in California and most other states, children could only legally have one mother—and father, for that matter. Such policies posed challenges to having the parental rights of both parents recognized, which also impinged on the rights of children born in same-sex unions. For example, when a lesbian couple had a child through donor insemination, the nonbiological mother—in states that allowed it—was legally required to formally adopt the child in order to be considered a legal parent. For heterosexual couples who had a child through donor insemination, the husband's role as a parent was legally and socially assumed. It was not until 2016 that changes in California law permitted the gender-neutral term *parent* on birth certificates, so that both partners of a same-sex couple could be listed as a child's parents. Until then, some lesbian couples would list the nonbiological mother on the "father" line and cross out the word *father*. Even when same-sex partners both have their names on their child's birth certificate, the nonbiological parent still does not necessarily have legal protection over his or her relationship with the child. Second-parent adoption was required in order to have the relationship legally protected.

For lesbian couples who wanted to adopt a child instead of one of them becoming pregnant, one woman was required to adopt the child first, and then the other had to go through the same process, requiring several home studies by caseworkers and a great deal of money spent on attorneys' fees. Heterosexual couples could adopt a child together without all these added obstacles, and the process only required one adoption procedure. Furthermore, the ability for the second same-sex parent to adopt varies from state to state, county to county, and court to court—and was subject to the whims of judges.

In addition, custody disputes between lesbian couples who separated after having children were typically decided in favor of the biological mother; in many states, this is still the case. Often, nonbiological mothers have been denied visitation—even if the couple started their family together—because second-parent adoption either was not available or was not recognized.

In some states—for example, California—same-sex couples were able to adopt (although, in 1995, then-governor Pete Wilson attempted to change this). This was not the case throughout most of the United States. In states that allowed second-parent adoptions, lesbian couples who had children together typically had to go through formalized adoption proceedings for the nonbiological mother so that she and the child had a legally protected relationship. This meant that the couple were required to open their home to caseworkers, hire adoption attorneys, spend a considerable amount of money for legal advice, and go to court in order to have the relationship between the nonbiological mother and child legally recognized.

Bonnie (thirty-nine) and Sharon (forty) each gave birth to a child by the same donor. I first interviewed them in 1992, at their home in Berkeley, before Bonnie knew she was pregnant with their first child, and I spoke with them again in 1997. Sharon delivered their second child prematurely in 1996. Their second child was a pound and a half at birth and remained in the hospital for several months, undergoing numerous diagnostic tests and surgeries before he could go home with his mothers. Bonnie and Sharon were at the hospital constantly, keeping vigil over their fragile infant and taking turns returning home to take care of their other child. They remarked on how wonderful the nurses and hospital staff were about recognizing them as a family, asking them both to make crucial medical decisions and sign necessary forms on the infant's behalf.

They told me about the process of having their family legally recognized through second-parent adoption:

BONNIE: The first time we went through the second-parent adoption it was like we needed to prove that this child is both of ours—we didn't totally feel like parents. By the second kid you just feel like people don't get this. Why deal with the public? Your life is busy—diapers and preschool—you can't feel more like a family than you do with two kids. Especially with all that we went through when our second child was born.

SHARON: It [second parent adoption] is something you need to do, but it's not like you need to prove anything to the world anymore. All you have to do is spend five minutes in our house to know we're a family.

BONNIE: So, the same social worker [from the first adoption] came to our house. The first time the process was really long. She asked us all these questions. She had to see us together, and separately, and each alone with the child, and so on. This time we were preparing, thinking she'd go through the same steps. Instead, she just used the visit to do her paperwork on our case. We had to have the whole family present, but she only asked us two questions and that was it.

SHARON: She talked to us both together, instead of separately. She told us it was better to have two children, and not just one, and then she left.

BONNIE: So, finally, we went to the court, and our daughter sat on the judge's lap while he signed the adoption papers. It's nice, she had this little signing experience. It's one little piece of the puzzle of putting together her family. It helps her make sense of how Sharon adopted her just like I adopted her brother.

While second-parent adoption worked for Bonnie and Sharon, it does not always—and lesbian couples are scrutinized by the state in ways straight couples are not. While many courts recognize it is in the child's best interest to receive the benefit of both parents, regardless of sexual orientation, others do not, thereby challenging the stability of same-sex couples and the children conceived in those unions and denying them basic rights that heterosexual couples and their children enjoy without scrutiny.

During the process of trying to conceive, what it means to be a mother rarely enters the picture. The focus is on the physical process itself, on choosing a donor and achieving a successful pregnancy. Once successful, though, the focus shifts. For example, the first time I interviewed Bonnie and Sharon, they were in the process of choosing the right donor and getting pregnant. When I interviewed them again several years later, they had completely forgotten about how they chose a sperm donor until I reminded them. What had once seemed so significant now barely entered their minds. Instead, their focus was on what it meant to be a family with two mothers, and how they experienced creating a family under nontraditional circumstances. Furthermore, they resented having to explain their family structure to those who "just don't get it."

CONCLUSION

Deciding to have a child through donor insemination is different for single women and lesbian couples. For couples, the decision to use a donor to have a child is similar to any couple's decision to start a family. The main issue is first deciding on the source of the sperm. For single women, the decision to use a donor is usually not their first choice. It comes with increasing age, fear that time is running out, and a certain amount of sadness at going it alone and not having found the right partner. Interestingly, both groups of women described having absent, fluctuating, or social rather than genetic fathers in their lives and expressed the perception that the presence of loving parents and extended family was more important than that of a biological father.

For lesbian couples that do conceive, having their families recognized posed a major challenge. On a federal level, same-sex couples were denied the right to marry until 2015. This means that same-sex couples that had children together could not exercise the same parental rights that heterosexual couples enjoyed without question. This had a devastating effect on children's rights as well, as courts routinely decided in favor of the biological mother at the expense of the other mother. Lesbian couples like Bonnie and Sharon attempted to work around these legal obstacles through second-parent adoption and by using the same donor so their children would be biological half siblings. Others have tried to level the parental playing field by having one partner donate eggs to the other partner to carry the child, so both moms could have some contribution to the child. But for lesbian couples, legal parenthood could never be taken for granted in the way it could for straight couples. This legal vulnerability also plays into how women choose a sperm donor; known donors are considered higher risk legally.

Women's decisions to conceive a child through donor insemination are rooted in a belief that a child can grow up healthy and well adjusted without a father (or father figure) in the household, as long as the child is loved and well cared for. This notion has been supported by research (Golombok 2015; Fulcher et al. 2006). For many women, the meanings of fatherhood are flexible and not always consistent with biological kinship. At the same time, while women do emphasize that a biological father is not necessary for a child to be well adjusted, most women also maintain that father figures are important to consider. A woman's, or a couple's, decision to use a known donor or an anonymous sperm bank donor is also connected to her own perceptions and experiences of men involved—or not—in her own childhood, as well as to her belief regarding whether the child will wish to have access to information about his or her biological father.

Ellen Lewin (1993) explores how the social role of motherhood influences a woman's self-definition regardless of sexual orientation, and finds many similarities between the experiences of lesbian and heterosexual single women. Even though sex and reproduction occur separately for the women in my study, motherhood, womanhood, and sexuality seem conflated for many of my informants in terms of their definitions of self. However, in discussing their emotional reactions to infertility, many lesbians have interpreted it as being linked to their sexual orientation, whereas heterosexual women have offered other explanations of self-blame. Although technologies have effectively separated reproduction from heterosexual intercourse, gender identity is still strongly connected to the ability to procreate: the meanings of motherhood and womanhood have been conflated for both groups. At the same time, although social fatherhood is prioritized over biological fatherhood when it comes to relationships, donors are selected based on a variety of social characteristics that are perceived as potentially heritable, just in case nature trumps nurture.

4 · SEMEN TRANSACTIONS

Donor Screening and the Regulation of Sexuality

UC Men, Get Paid for What You're Already Doing!
—Sperm bank advertisement in the *Daily Cal,* 1991

I was sitting at the front desk at The Sperm Bank of California, in Berkeley, entering my data on their computer. A sandy-haired man, most likely in his early twenties, seemed somewhat uneasy—and in fact turned red—as he approached the counter. I imagined he was probably a first-time sperm donor and mistook me for the receptionist. He stumbled while trying to find the appropriate words to refer to a sexual act that was, in this context, part of a clinical practice to provide a product: "Is this where I go to make a deposit? Or, uh, what's the term, 'provide a specimen'?"

This type of interaction happens daily in most sperm banks, but for the men who "make deposits," or "provide specimens," there is often at least a small hint of embarrassment. It struck me at this moment that the way in which semen is collected—obviously through male masturbation—is disguised behind the medically and economically veiled language of deposits, specimens, and samples, which rarely addresses the experiences of the men who "donate" or how those samples are retrieved.

The university newspaper advertisement featured in this chapter's epigraph— "Get Paid for What You're Already Doing"—is a tongue-in-cheek way of making the linkages between sexual performance and income explicit, and it is designed to grab prospective donors' attention. Sperm donor advertisements are rife with innuendo; eye-catching imagery of young, handsome men; and humor: "Inside every hero there are millions more," "Sperm donation: more fun than giving blood," and "Are you up for it?" How sexuality is presented, perceived, managed, and regulated throughout the sperm bank industry intersects with men's motivations and experiences as sperm bank donors.

Numerous contradictions exist in regard to semen and its collection. In her book *Sperm Counts*, Lisa Jean Moore (2007) explores the multiple meanings of semen and sperm and argues that how sperm is defined depends on one's vantage point and the social context. Semen's meaning when viewed under a laboratory microscope is very different from its meaning at a crime scene, for a sex worker, or for a romantic lover. For heterosexual couples, the partners' relationship to semen and sperm will shift according to whether they are trying to conceive or trying to avoid conception. Women who enjoy sex with men may view donor semen differently from women who have sex with women—many of whom report being "grossed out" by having to handle semen while trying to inseminate their partners.

Sexuality is simultaneously present and absent, sanitized in a professional, clinical setting. Semen itself can be construed as both gift and commodity. It is thought to contain and transmit various social, as well as genetic, traits, which are assigned value and meaning, resulting in a very convoluted interpretation of heritability. Semen can contain and transmit both positive and negative elements: sperm is necessary for a woman to achieve a pregnancy, yet the fluid that contains it can also put a woman at risk for contracting sexually transmitted diseases, including HIV/AIDS. It can also be a vehicle for transmitting genetic diseases to future offspring if donors are not sufficiently screened. Various contradictions surround semen collection and transaction, including the presence, absence, regulation, and management of donor sexuality within the sperm bank industry. Sperm bank staff are charged with containing a messy substance, freezing it, storing it, and shipping it to clients around the world.

The tensions around semen exchange and sexuality can be seen in various domains: at the level of state and national policies that regulate screening procedures and storage policies at tissue-banking facilities; in the reproductive industry and social engineering; in the policies and philosophies of individual sperm banks; and in the individual men who provide sperm and the people who purchase it. In each of these domains, perceptions of male sexuality and notions of risk influence who can and cannot become a sperm donor. In his work on HIV/AIDS, Paul Farmer (1992) notes a "geography of blame," where Haitians, hemophiliacs, and homosexuals are perceived as responsible for the spread of HIV. This geography of blame enters into the realm of sperm donation as well and informs Food and Drug Administration guidelines concerning who is permitted to become a sperm donor. Since men who have sex with men are considered a "high-risk group," they are, for all intents and purposes, disqualified from becoming sperm donors.

Not only does sexuality influence who can become a donor, but once a man becomes a sperm donor, his sexual activity comes under the scrutiny of the clinic. Men with sexual partners and men who masturbate outside the parameters of sperm donation do not make good donors because these activities reduce the quality and quantity of sperm in the semen. This chapter links the perceptions and management of sexuality with the market in reproductive technologies and genetic material while focusing on how philosophies surrounding reproduction are played out in regard to national health regulations and individual sperm bank policies. The men who provide semen intersect with the broader regulatory policies of the state and sperm bank practices.

The myriad symbolic meanings of semen exist at several levels: at the sperm bank where semen is collected, analyzed, tested, washed, looked at under a microscope, frozen, thawed, assessed for sperm content, frozen again, cataloged, stored, and sold; among the women who peruse the donor profiles to find out more about its source, discuss it, assign comparative value to it, purchase it, drive it around in their cars, take it home, thaw it, insert it, purchase more, store it in a sperm bank for later use, and construct identities about the men who provided it; and at the level of social mores, which prompt debates about the "morality" of its collection and sale. Sperm banks are businesses that deal in semen on a daily basis. Their screening procedures are affected by government regulations and health policies—specifically in regard to the reduction of risk for transmission of HIV/AIDS and other communicable diseases. Male heteronormative sexuality is managed both within and outside the walls of sperm banks as a mechanism for managing "risk." Although Rainbow Flag Health Services (RFHS) actively recruited gay male donors for lesbian and bisexual clients, it also managed the risks and regulated the behavior of donors, though in a more sex-positive atmosphere, as will be described in this chapter.

THE CONTENTS OF SEMEN

Sperm refers to the actual cells contained within the ejaculate, or semen. At sperm banks, semen (containing millions of sperm cells) is collected, purchased, frozen, and sold. It is usually a single sperm cell that fertilizes a woman's egg and results in a pregnancy. If a prospective donor produces a sample that has a low sperm count (for example, due to recent sexual activity) or low motility (movement), it will usually be rejected.

Anthropological studies on masculinity explore the symbolic meanings of semen and reveal how, cross-culturally, semen is interpreted as containing the essence of masculine identity and power. Gilbert Herdt's (1981) work on "semen transactions" among the Sambia in New Guinea, for example, addresses the tribe's practice in which boys approaching manhood must acquire semen from older men in order to become men themselves. Joseph Alter (1997) addresses male celibacy in India and the cultural anxieties surrounding sex, semen, health, and male identity. Lawrence Cohen explores "the reification of 'semen loss' as a cultural truth" and the "every day excess of seminal exchange" in India (1999, 113). He examines the dynamics at play when rural (strong) men sell their semen to urban (weak) men and identifies how such practices result in a transmission of power and strength. Cohen's informant states, "These city boys . . . they come with their fathers' money and I give them something. They take my strength [referring to his semen] and I take some money" (1999, 113).

This body of work not only points to the cultural complexity of meanings surrounding semen and its exchange but also brings to the fore how the perceptions of semen quality affect its economic value. This both reveals how perceived semen quality can be translated into monetary value and highlights the parallels between the sexual exchange of semen and the economic exchange of semen between donors and the sperm bank industry. Semen transactions in the U.S. sperm bank industry are, of course, very different from those among the Sambia or in India. Within the sperm bank walls, these transactions are imbued with different social meanings and are connected to clinical practice rather than homoerotic social relations.

Masculinity and sexuality are also linked in the sperm donation process, and masturbation is contained in the clinical setting. In her research on masculinity and masturbation in men's experiences with infertility treatment, Marcia Inhorn (2007b) correctly asserts that in infertility research, and among feminist scholars focusing on assisted reproduction, men's embodiment, including the often-embarrassing process of providing sperm, is often downplayed, while women's embodied experiences receive primary attention. For sperm donors, a process that is initially embarrassing—due the inherent sexuality involved in giving samples—eventually becomes routine (Tober 2002). As others similarly note, donating semen involves an "embodiment of masculinity and male sexuality" that is managed in clinical and laboratory spaces (Mohr 2016, 323).

The sperm bank industry and the market for donor sperm are both heavily influenced by the notion that some traits—social or physical—are more desirable than others, and that these traits reside in the sperm. Semen is a vehicle for the transmission of genetic material (and genetic diseases) and carries various complex meanings—biological, evolutionary, historical, cultural, political, technological, and sexual. Widely shared perceptions of genetic inheritance, in both the scientific and lay communities, profoundly affect how genetic material (of which sperm is but one type) is selected for "donation" and how this material is marketed and exchanged. These perceptions of heritability, with sperm as a transmitter of genetic material, shape the ways in which potential donors are screened and their semen sold. Indeed, these notions of what sperm contains, coupled with cultural values surrounding the reproduction of certain types of individuals over others, affects the entire market for human gametes.

SEXUALITY, HIV/AIDS, AND SPERM BANK REGULATIONS

> The state of New York has regulations that say that a sperm bank cannot even be in receipt—much less store the sperm—of any man who has had sex with another man since 1977. Most sperm banks [in the country] have a New York state license because they ship sperm into New York, and they use that as one of their reasons for not accepting gay men as donors. So, what they're saying is in order to protect their profits, they are willing to go along with these bigoted regulations of the state of New York. I find no moral justification for that.   —Leland, RFHS[1]

Masculinity and sexuality are managed throughout the sperm donation process, both in terms of who can become a sperm donor and in terms of the daily management of sexual activities in order to produce quality semen samples with abundant, strong-swimming sperm. In most sperm banks, donors are required to be heterosexual and have limited sexual partners. The management of donor sexuality serves dual purposes: to maintain both the quality and the safety of the product.

Aside from transmitting genetic material found in sperm, semen also contains the potential to transmit disease. The HIV/AIDS epidemic has had a dramatic impact on the sperm bank industry. Leland explained to me how the entire industry was shut down for six months in 1982, when the HIV/AIDS crisis first struck. During this period, the Centers for Disease Control (CDC) and the Health Department were trying to figure out how to stop the spread of AIDS, as well as how to regulate the sperm bank industry to eliminate the risk of HIV transmission for recipients of donor semen.

Once the blood test for HIV became available, potential donors were given mandatory HIV tests (as well as being screened for other diseases) and their semen was then quarantined for six months, at which point they were retested for HIV. If both HIV tests were negative, their cryopreserved semen could then be sold to recipients. The CDC and the American Association of Tissue Banks recommended homosexuals be banned from sperm banks, because they were in a perceived high-risk group for HIV—despite the fact that heterosexual men are not immune to HIV, some men who have sex with men might not consider themselves "homosexual" (or may not truthfully answer the question), and adequate screening measures are in place to ensure that men who test HIV positive do not become sperm donors.

Many states require that a sperm bank be a member of the American Association of Tissue Banks. This means the bank must subscribe to the CDC guidelines that bar gay men from being anonymous sperm donors because they are in a "high-risk" group for HIV/AIDS. The degree to which CDC guidelines are implemented varies between states and between sperm banks. The states of New

York and Maryland, for example, have some of the strictest regulations in the country surrounding the shipment of semen. As Leland noted, any tissue or sperm bank that ships semen to these states cannot even be in receipt of the sperm of any man who has admitted to having sex with another man since 1977. In 2005 the Food and Drug Administration passed a regulation barring any man who has had sex with a man in the past five years from becoming an anonymous sperm donor. "Directed" donors—a donor whom the intended mother knows and chooses—do not fall under this restriction.

Aside from New York and Maryland, very few states have regulations barring gay men from being sperm donors outright. These regulations obviously affect the way in which sperm banks are able to conduct their business, especially when part of that business involves buying and selling semen. Leland's business for gay sperm was geographically limited because he rejected the New York regulations, and he was not a member of the American Association of Tissue Banks. The CDC guidelines, though not uniformly implemented from state to state, demonstrate how a "geography of blame" (Farmer 1992) can influence a "geography of reproduction"—placing social and geographic limitations on who can reproduce and where.

Robert became a donor at RFHS after having been rejected at another sperm bank for his sexual orientation. He contacted me in 2000, after seeing a flyer for my study at RFHS. Shortly thereafter, we met at a small Vietnamese restaurant near the Berkeley campus: "I understand why most sperm banks screen out gay men. People are concerned and cautious about exposure risks to diseases. I figured the recipients are going to want to know, so I had to be honest on the intake form. I thought they at least had the right to know as much as they can. But in some way I feel that when it comes to parenting, people have the right to choose their criteria even if, in my view, it's irrational."

Several informants in the sperm bank industry discussed the impact these state regulations have had on their businesses. As Leland pointed out, most local sperm banks have a New York license that permits them to ship semen to clients in that state. This means that a sperm bank in California, for example, that ships semen to clients in New York cannot accept semen from a gay man for any reason. It cannot store the semen of gay men who wish to pay for sperm storage, nor can it accept recipients who wish to use a known, or directed, donor who is gay. As Leland states, "Some in the industry question whether these regulations exist in the interest of public safety or if they are another form of social engineering. There is no scientific reason that would protect the public, to justify preventing gay or bisexual men from being sperm donors. Any justification you could have in using the criteria for blood donations goes out the window for sperm donation because of the quarantine period. You can't freeze blood."

Regulations banning certain groups of men from becoming sperm donors because they belong to a perceived "high-risk" category for certain communicable diseases may seem to be a logical remedy to a realistic public health concern. In this example, the concern regarding what is contained in the *semen* is collapsed with a concern regarding what is contained in the *sperm*. Are these policies really about the risk of transmitting HIV/AIDS, or are they connected to larger social or eugenic concerns regarding the heritability of homosexuality, or "gay genes"? The notion of risk is coupled with the problem of social engineering. Can the regulations banning gay men as semen donors actually be construed as a means to regulate sexuality? How are our notions of sexuality—particularly gay male sexuality—linked to cultural ideas of promiscuity, recklessness, and risk, as well as to concerns about the potential genetic basis of homosexuality?

Jonathon described his own experience as a gay man who applied to be a donor at several sperm banks. I asked him about the interviews they conducted to screen him as a donor and whether they asked him about his sexual orientation. He responded, "No. They would never say straight out, but it seemed like very quickly the interview would come to a close with them. And I asked about that and they said they won't say it, but they aren't interested."

These restrictions only apply in instances when men reveal their sexual practices to the repository in question. Trust is important between sperm banks and their donors. Sperm banks have various mechanisms by which they establish trust between themselves and their donors—including a lengthy screening process that involves various medical exams and tests for sexually transmitted diseases, as well as more socially based methods of screening, including questionnaires and personal interviews. This notion of trust also enters into the debate surrounding financial remuneration of semen donors.

BECOMING A DONOR

Men have a range of motivations for becoming sperm donors. One of the most common reasons, what brings them to the sperm bank in the first place, is usually the promise of financial compensation. There is a lengthy screening process that potential donors have to go through before they can become donors, so those who are purely doing it for the money, or need money right away, are often screened out at the outset. Judy Garvey, who at one time handled donor screening at The Sperm Bank of California (TSBC), told me about their initial screening process:

> Most men call up to find out if they can be a sperm donor and what the requirements are. When I tell them about the screening process, that it takes a couple of months before they can start, and we want them to commit to a year, some of the guys say, "That's too big a commitment for me." And I respect that. We find that works in our favor because then we have donors who are willing to have delayed gratification when it comes to money, and we know they are committed

to being a donor because of what it gives to someone else. Anyone who says, "I want money now. Pay me now," they're desperate for this, but the other guys make better donors because they're committed.

We also screen a lot of guys out because of their backgrounds and their sex lives. For their background, we don't want guys who use drugs and alcohol, because that can lead to bad sexual judgment. How can you be sure they're practicing safe sex when they're smashed out of their minds? We also can't accept gay men here, which is a shame because a lot of women, especially our lesbian clients, want gay sperm. And then there are guys we turn away because of the number of sexual partners, like they have way too many partners and they don't know anything about their partners' sexual histories.

As Judy revealed, while most men decide to become donors because they need the money, there is a point at which a donor's desire for compensation decreases his suitability as a donor. Likewise, while all TSBC's donors are presumably heterosexual, hyperheterosexuality—having too many sexual partners or engaging in risky behaviors—can also disqualify a donor. The clinic wants men who are committed to the process, are responsible, and are easy to work with over an extended period of time. Ideally, even though a prospective donor may need and seek financial compensation, he should also be motivated by other considerations.

Jake, twenty-five, is a software engineer in Palo Alto. He was a junior in college at Stanford University when he first found out about sperm donation from a roommate. He was raised in a strict Catholic household in the Midwest and went to private Catholic school up through high school, but he eventually rejected his Catholic upbringing. He told me about how his decision to become a sperm donor was a combination of needing money and rebellion against his conservative upbringing:

JAKE: My roommate told me he was doing this donor gig and he was getting paid thirty-five bucks a shot. I said, "Wow!" I was blown away. Being from the Midwest I never imagined anyone would pay for my sperm. I was shocked and I thought it was funny, but the more I thought about it, I mean, if you're healthy and stuff, why not? I wanted to do it while I was in college because I needed money, but I didn't have a car to get up there, to the sperm bank.

DIANE: So what did you like about the idea?

JAKE: Part of it, honestly, [was that] I wasn't fond of the religious upbringing I had. I was really opposed to Catholicism and organized religion. So being a sperm donor is sort of my private little joke. It's like, "Ha, ha, ha, Catholic Church." This is an alternative way of making family, single women and lesbians, as opposed to the man-woman central tenet of Catholicism. It's my way of saying "screw you" to the Catholic Church.

DIANE: So what was it like for you the first time you donated?

JAKE: I was definitely a little embarrassed—very shy to go in there. But I thought, "Well, I just need to do it and see how it is." So I was kind of shaky, but the guy who worked there actually seemed more embarrassed than I was. So that was kind of funny. But now it's just routine.

It's kinda funny though. I just happened to look at their website the other day, and I looked up my donor number, and there's a box checked that says I have a successful pregnancy. That kind of blew me away. Maybe I was in denial, but I thought there was no way anyone would ever buy my sperm. Now at least I know if I got hit by a truck or something at least there's biological DNA that's mine out there. That's kind of nice to know.

Jake's decision to become a donor was motivated by a couple of factors: financial need and a kind of cosmic joke at the expense of the Catholic Church. He also addressed the element of sexuality and his embarrassment at having to masturbate at the clinic for the first time, embarrassment that was shared by the sperm bank staff. When he first became a donor, he did not really think about the people who would be receiving his sperm, or the children that could be produced from it, saying he was "in denial" that someone would actually choose him. Learning that there had been a successful pregnancy from his donations gave him a different perspective: it simultaneously alleviated his sense of reproductive responsibility and increased his curiosity, causing him to hope that someday he might meet the children born from his sperm. When I asked him how he felt when he found out he had at least one child out there, he said, "It makes me feel good to know I made these people happy. They have a kid now. And I could have this little surprise down the road of someone contacting me. That would be kind of fun."

Some men initially look into sperm donation both because of the compensation and because they are familiar with the struggles people face when confronted with infertility. Ricardo, a thirty-five-year-old Filipino American, was recently divorced when he first looked into sperm donation in 1995. Although he needed money, his initial reasons for becoming a donor were more personal:

My sister and her husband were having problems getting pregnant. Seeing her struggle and all that she went through to finally have my niece made me feel like I wanted to give back—to help someone else have a baby—because that struggle is so profound. They really went through a lot.

So I had been thinking about it, but I was married at the time, and my wife didn't really support the idea. A year or so later, my wife and I separated, so there were a lot of financial problems. I bought a house in Oakland at the height of the market in 1990, and when we were separating, we couldn't sell the property. So it was really rough. I was scrambling to get a cup of coffee.

And then one day I saw an ad in the *East Bay Express*, and it sort of all came together. I needed the money. It was something I had wanted to do for a while, to help someone else. And I didn't have to worry anymore about what my wife would think. So I contacted the sperm bank.

Ricardo's motivations were a mix of altruism and a need for money. If he had not needed the money, he would have been a donor purely to help other people, since he understood what it was like to go through infertility from his sister's experience. Some men are also motivated by a desire to pass on their genes, and may perceive themselves as exceptional. For example, Don, twenty-eight, thought it was his social responsibility to enhance the gene pool: "I played baseball since I was five. I've been athletic all my life. I'm fit. I'm working on a masters in economics at a great university. And I think I've got great genes and I need to pass them on. Sperm donation helps me do that. I hope the kids enjoy my genes as much as I have."

Men have a range of reasons for becoming sperm bank donors. While financial compensation usually plays into that decision, there are other factors as well, such as a desire to help or to achieve genetic continuation. Men's motivations may also change throughout the process: someone who first looked into it for financial reasons may find himself continuing to be a sperm donor even when he no longer needs the money, because he believes in the cause. Also, when donors discover that children have been born from their donations, their perspectives may shift with the realization that there are actual people out in the world who are inheritors of their DNA. Decisions are complex and change over time.

SCREENING, FREEZING, AND COUNTING SPERM

All sperm banks use the same basic procedures for screening and freezing semen and counting sperm, in accordance with CDC guidelines designed to minimize risk. Semen sold through a sperm bank must be frozen and quarantined for six months. Before 1982, women were typically able to purchase fresh semen, which many believed was more potent than frozen semen. But fresh semen is no longer available at most sperm banks. Women who use directed donors—men they know or meet through various networks—typically want to use fresh semen. But not all medical providers will do a fresh insemination; the sperm provider is also the woman's sexual partner. Directed donors are still usually tested for the same communicable diseases as sperm bank donors, at the request of the women who decide to use them. Before the HIV/AIDS crisis, fresh semen could also be obtained through many fertility clincs. But most private practices would not inseminate single women or lesbian couples—this was especially true in the 1990s and in many places is still true today.

Before a potential donor is accepted into a sperm bank program, various medical tests must be done to ensure he is free from a variety of diseases, including HIV 1 and HIV 2, HTLV 1 and 2 (a virus thought to cause certain types of leukemia), hepatitis B and C, cytomegalovirus (CMV), syphilis, gonorrhea, streptococcus, chlamydia, and a variety of others. These tests are conducted on blood samples, semen samples, urine samples, and urethral cultures. Some banks also conduct genetic testing for Tay-Sachs disease, cystic fibrosis, and other genetic disorders. The entire screening process takes approximately six to eight weeks, during which time the semen is quarantined. Potential donors who have passed these medical screening tests are retested at the end of six months for HIV, HTLV, CMV, herpes, and syphilis, and every six months thereafter. Donors' sperm is simultaneously screened for how well it survives the freezing process. Fewer than 11 percent of applicants are eventually accepted as donors. If a donor passes all of these tests, at the end of six months his semen is made available for purchase. The ability to screen, count, and catalog sperm samples is important in terms of minimizing medical risk, increasing the likelihood of clients' achieving pregnancy, and also ensuring clients receive the product they purchased.

Leland took me on a tour of his facility while going about his daily work, and explained what he looks for in prospective donors' sperm. Looking through a microscope at a semen sample, he explained:

I looked around, and I wasn't counting the moving cells, I was counting the dead ones, because you can't count them when they're moving. You count them when they're not moving. The state doesn't like it when I call them dead. "There's no proof those cells were dead, there's only proof that they were not moving."

Yes, they were not moving, presumed dead. I first counted the not-moving cells, and now I'm going to freeze them in such a way that none of them will survive and, then we can count all of them. Then we can subtract the previously not-moving ones from the total number. That will give us the total number of previously moving cells so we can figure out the guy's sperm count per cc. A guy has to have a pretty good sperm count to be a donor, but you're also looking at the shape of the sperm and how they move.

The screening process at sperm banks, however, does not only concern the physical and medical characteristics of the donor, his semen, and his sperm. The screening process also involves questions about sexual behavior. Leland explained how donors are screened each time they provide a specimen:

This is one of our established donors. Every time he donates semen, I ask him, When was the last time you ejaculated? "Four days ago." Was any of your ejaculation spilled? "No." Did you have sex with someone who is not your regular partner since the last time you donated? "No." Have you come into contact with any infectious diseases since the last time you donated? "No." Do you have any unusual discharge from your penis, or any sores on your penis, or any rashes on your body? "No." And, section B, do you have a regular partner that you have told us about? This should be yes, not no. I ask him these rather than have him fill it out. If yes, is he the only person you had sex with? Are you the only person he/she has had sex with? Is your partner HIV negative?

Leland asks these same questions every time a man donates, and he can decide not to sell his sperm depending on how the donor answers the questions. This line of questioning, at this level of graphic detail regarding one's sexual behavior, is not typical of other sperm banks. Because Leland's donors are almost exclusively men who have sex with men, he finds it prudent to ask details about sexual behavior. As he points out, he does this despite the fact that "we have a test that's as close to perfect as humanly possible [for detecting HIV]," so we "don't have to worry about lifestyle, and we don't need to discriminate on the basis of sexual orientation."

After being screened out of a number of other sperm banks, Jonathon, like Robert, also became a Rainbow Flag donor. I asked Jonathon how his sex life outside the sperm bank was affected by his work as a donor, and what the screening process was like for him:

JONATHON: Each time I went in I had to keep records of everything, every activity I think, what happened with whom, and then I would report it before each donation. I mean they asked questions like, "Did you put your penis in someone's mouth? Did someone put their penis in yours?" You know, for every sexual body part. I wasn't doing anything, so it wasn't too hard for me to fill out. And two and a half months for me is not a big deal for no sex. But no physical closeness, that is a little hard. So I wouldn't do anything that was even a gray area.

DIANE: Not even oral sex?

JONATHON: No, no.

HANDLING SEXUALITY

Male masturbation is obviously necessary for collecting semen, but in many sperm banks, sexuality, whether in the form of erotic material or even daily discourse, is glaringly absent from the repository atmosphere itself. In all the interviews I conducted at sperm banks, I never once heard the word *masturbation*. The act was instead referred to as "it."

The fact that masturbation is never discussed directly, even though it is necessary in order to obtain a semen sample, implies a certain uneasiness with the process—an attempt to maintain clinical distance by removing the element of sexuality. How masturbation is managed without discussion provides insight into the tensions donors and clinicians experience in regard to this element of male sexuality, as well as indicating a moral problem of pleasure (Foucault 1990).

The ways in which sexuality is both present and absent in the sperm banks provide insight into how sexuality is constructed and controlled. Each sperm bank has different policies regarding how male sexuality is to be handled. They are linked—in part—to a concern regarding the transmission of sexually transmitted diseases, including HIV/AIDS. However, even personal values surrounding sexuality—for example, the use of erotic material for inducing arousal—influence the policies of sex in sperm banks differently.

At TSBC, the policies regarding erotic material are strict for sperm donors but less restrictive for men who are paying for sperm storage, according to Barbara.

> We have three rooms here, where men provide semen—whether he's one of our donors or a man who is actually paying for the service of sperm storage. We try to create a comfortable environment that's not too sterile looking and not too clinical, but that's professional and comfortable at the same time.
>
> Our policy is that we don't provide any literature for sexual stimulation. However, we also understand there are some men who have an impossible time. It's not so much the donors, but the men who come in for sperm storage who have this problem. . . . If he is a private donor, he can bring his own literature but he can't leave it. He has to take it with him. . . .
>
> Also, I think that the donors are more in the habit. . . . I think there's already a certain comfort level with it, or they wouldn't be interested in being donors in the first place.

Barbara makes a distinction between two types of men who provide semen to the sperm bank: paid donors and men who are there to pay for sperm storage services (usually because they have a medical condition and are receiving treatment for it that could render them infertile). Policies surrounding sexuality and sexual literature vary depending on whether one is a donor or a customer of the sperm bank. It is assumed that donors are accustomed to engaging in masturbation, or other sexual activity, almost anywhere and without need for erotic stimulation. This implies a sort of wanton sexuality that becomes managed and regulated when men decide to become donors.

Men who have been providing sperm for a while share this perception of sexuality. Jonathon described his own experience.

> I wasn't embarrassed at all. You know, I think it's a very, very small number of men who have trouble with masturbating. I think it's kind of natural to everybody. And physiologically, whether you masturbate or not your body continually produces

sperm and it can't hold an unending volume. If it does, you need to see a surgeon. But I do realize from the history it was once believed the man contained little, tiny, completely formed babies and just deposited them in the woman, fully formed. And it wasn't until recently it was understood that the mother and the father both contribute. But I can understand where if they thought each of those was a fully formed human that masturbation would be wasting seed, but it's not really a seed yet. It's half a seed.

At RFHS, male sexuality appeared to be much more readily accepted than at any of the other sperm banks I visited. Leland showed me the room "where men go to provide their specimens." I looked around and saw the kind of examining table one would see in any gynecologist's office, complete with stirrups and white tissue paper that lined the table's surface. The room looked as if it had once been a bedroom. A VCR and television, homosexual pornographic videotapes, and similar magazines were placed within a couple of feet of the examining table. Leland explained, "This is where we do the inseminations. As you can see, we have material to help men ejaculate. We have a VCR and a television. We have videos and printed material. Although, on occasion I have been asked by some of my gay donors if I could help them and I had to very politely say, 'Thank you very much, I appreciate the compliment, but that's not the ethical thing to do. No, I just can't do that, thank you very much.'"

As I surveyed this room and listened to Leland speak, the way in which reproduction occurred in this room suddenly struck me as a bit odd. It was room that was at one time a bedroom and was now a place where men went to masturbate and women went to inseminate, representing a merging of male solitary sexuality and female reproductivity apart from heterosexual intercourse. This was a singular space in which pornography was viewed in order to produce a product and technology was used to produce a pregnancy—sex and reproduction, two activities now devoid of intimate human contact. In this one space, sexual acts were occurring and babies were being made, but there was no contact between the men performing sexual acts and the women who were trying to conceive children. The only connection between the man and the woman was Leland, the person who collected the semen and later transferred it into the woman. A room simultaneously outfitted for gynecological exams and pornographic pleasure connects sexuality and reproduction in a very nontraditional way indeed.

I asked Leland what he thought about banks that do not permit pornographic materials. He responded,

> I think that's so rude. It seems ridiculous to deny any type of sexuality—you have to have some type of sexuality to get the product. You have to have something. I also heard that at one sperm bank they send you to the bathroom. I thought, "Oh, come on. Please be nice." I mean, these guys are helping people out.

It's also true that when a man is sexually stimulated he will produce a higher volume and a higher concentration of sperm. I've been saying that for years and everyone thought I was crazy. Recently, there was a paper at the American Fertility Society. They looked at men with low sperm counts, without any pornography, and then they had them come back a week later, and showed them pornographic videos and got much better samples. Seems reasonable to me. We get turned on; we produce more.

At Rainbow Flag, Leland had a view of male sexuality and fertility that is not necessarily shared by personnel at other sperm banks. He viewed the proposition from the donor asking for "help" as a compliment, stated his position that it was not ethical, and allowed the man to provide his sample alone. When potential donors made similar comments at TSBC, they were perceived as inappropriate and the men were rejected as donors. RFHS appeared to have a more relaxed stance on male sexuality—gay, straight, or otherwise—than sperm banks founded and run by women.

Leland also declared that to deny men access to pornography, or to require them to provide their samples in the bathroom, is "not being nice" to the men, who are "helping people out." For him, to reject this aspect of male sexuality is disrespectful, even dehumanizing. But for Barbara, the restriction against pornography is connected to her personal stance on the objectification of women. For Leland, as a gay man, porn—or the sexual objectification of men—is intended for erotic stimulation to deliver a quality product. This idea of "helping donors" ejaculate is not only found on sperm bank premises but also is popular in clinical sperm donor masturbation fantasies and depictions of sexual acts that can be found online. For example, a photo of attractive Chinese "sperm bank workers" dressed in clinical garb and serving an assembly line of "sperm donors" in a sterile clinical setting is just one representation of sex and sperm bank fantasies—in this case, it is the women who are performing "reproductive sex work" for men who apparently do not have hands (https://www.allsingaporestuff.com/article/man-dies-sperm-bank-after-4th-sperm-donation-10-days). Although the photo was later determined to be a hoax, and female sperm bank workers were not really helping donors with their "collection," it still speaks to the pornographic imaginary surrounding sperm donor life.

Another site contains a video of a man going to the front desk of a sperm bank, where an attractive woman nurse hands him a glass for his deposit. He goes back to an exam room, peruses one pornographic magazine after another, and is unable to get himself aroused enough to ejaculate. Frustrated, he leaves the room, feeling defeated until he sees another magazine on a table in the hallway. He rushes back into the exam room, emerges triumphant and refreshed, and places his sample on the counter in front of the nurse. She looks down at the magazine he had and longingly, with supple lips parted, looks at the photograph of a motorcycle (Aprilia n.d.). The advertisement depicts, in a humorous way, both the anxieties and frustration of providing sperm on demand, as well as communicating the idea that the company's motorcycle is more arousing than pornography featuring women. This is especially interesting in light of the fact that at least one of the donors I interviewed, Jake, told me he became a sperm donor because he wanted to buy a motorcycle, thereby exchanging one type of commodity for another. Sex, pornography, and product are linked both in the act of providing sperm and in the hypermasculine fantasy of winding through country roads, dressed in leathers, with a slick, two-hundred-horsepower machine roaring between one's legs.

SELLING SEMEN AND DISCIPLINARY PRACTICES OF SEX

Men who sell their semen are involved in a type of bodywork in which their ability to bring themselves to climax results in increased financial (or social or genetic) opportunities. The classified ads in the local University of California campus newspapers for The Sperm Bank of California enticed many men: "Get Paid for Something You're Already Doing." The fact that the specifics of the transaction—masturbation in exchange for money—are implied in the ad, rather than explicitly stated, points to the moral contradictions of sex in an industry where helping people create families is the main goal.

Men who work as sperm donors can make enough money to pay their rent or other expenses. Sean, who was a donor at an East Bay fertility clinic from 1987 to 1997, calculated that he made more money per hour as a sperm donor than he did as a software consulting contractor, for which he charged fifty dollars per hour. Sean considered sperm donation to be an easy and quick way of earning an income to supplement his work as a consultant: "It was just like a job. It's tedious; it's not at all exciting. And sometimes they'd call me back the next day after I had just given a sample, because some Joe had just canceled on them and the woman was coming in two hours to be inseminated. And it was like, 'Oh God, I've got to go jerk off again. Oh well, fifty bucks is fifty bucks.'"

Another man, Robert, a donor at Rainbow Flag, saw sperm donation as a way to be a parent as a gay man: "I'd always wanted to have kids growing up and it was a big conflict being gay, because I didn't want to marry a woman. I think that's really unfair to the woman. Since I'll be able to meet any child when they're three months old, this seemed like the best way for me to have kids in some way and be involved in their lives."

Sperm donation requires a donor to regulate his own sexuality, but this occurs to varying degrees. Robert told me how he decided to stop being a donor when he became interested in pursuing a sexual relationship with another man: "I started seeing someone and I was getting to the point where I wanted to start having sex again. So I talked to Leland about it and he and I both decided that if I was going to start having sex with a new partner, I should probably quit being a donor, so that's what I did."

For many donors, including Robert, there is an emphasis on controlling one's sexual behaviors involving other people while working as a donor. The ability to regulate and control sexual desires is important for many donors, both for financial reasons (donors who get paid receive no compensation for poor samples) and for ethical reasons, such as reducing the risk of contracting and transmitting sexually transmitted diseases. Robert had been rejected at other sperm banks before coming to RFHS. He had always wanted to be a dad, and he decided on this sperm bank because he would be able to meet the kid and the mother or mothers. This provided intrinsic motivation to adhere to the regulations on his sexual behavior. Not all donors limit their sexual partners, however, but they do regulate their sexual activity with those partners.

Chuck, forty, who was a donor at a private clinic between 1982 and 1984, when he was in his thirties, described how he regulated his sexual activity while also working as a sperm donor:

> This was the eighties, so they didn't have, really, much in the way of screening. I had a lot of different lovers at the time and some of them knew about my work as a donor and some of them didn't. But the ones who knew realized if I had to provide the next day they could get me just to the edge, as long as I didn't cross over. For women I'd just met, though, I didn't really feel comfortable telling them that tomorrow I had an appointment to beat off for twenty-five dollars.
>
> So I had about six relationships going on at the same time, but no one-night stands. And the doctor, this urologist, didn't seem to care. He would just farm these guys out to different gynecologists. He would call me up and say, "Oh, what are you doing tomorrow? Can we get a sample?" I was doing odd jobs at the time, so I was pretty much available on call. And the deal was you weren't supposed to have had an orgasm for two days. So I told him, "That's only eight hours' warning." So he said, "Well, when was the last time you had sex?" And it was last night. But he said, "Don't worry. You've always got a good sperm count, and this woman is ready to go and you're the only game in town."
>
> So I would just go there, get paid. They'd write me a check right away. And he told me the women, they'd ask for someone who looked like their husbands, or they'd say, "I want somebody Serbian." Now I'm Irish and sure as hell not Serbian, so who knows if they got what they wanted?

Chuck, who had been a donor before the HIV/AIDS crisis, had much more flexibility in terms of the screening process and his sexuality than did donors after the rise of HIV. While his sexual relationships were not scrutinized, he did control his body to avoid orgasm before his scheduled donation appointments. For the times he was called to provide outside of his scheduled appointments, the doctor relaxed his rules. Unlike most other donors I interviewed, Chuck felt his work as a donor had very little impact on his other sexual activities, aside from regulating when and where he would ejaculate.

As touched on earlier, the connection between sex work and sperm donation can, oddly, be a source of erotic fantasy. As I was researching sperm banks on the internet, one site came up that made a rather blatant connection between donor sexuality and the sex industry.[2] This page provided some informational links for sperm donors, but it primarily furnished links to a variety of pornographic websites, including "live females" performing sex acts over the internet and other sexual fantasies involving teens, black women, Asian women, lesbians, gay men, sadomasochism, and so on. This site also included alleged hidden-camera pictures of a man masturbating (or working) in a "masturbation room" at a "sperm bank." Here, the sperm bank becomes the site of voyeuristic and exhibitionist masturbation fantasies in which the "sperm donor" is the eroticized subject. Lower on the page it stated, "Remember, you can help other people by giving sperm!" And, "If you already have experiences visiting a sperm bank, please feel free to (anonymously) tell about it."

Men's sperm bank stories were solicited to become the topic of sexual fantasy, but the hint of altruism, of helping others, is still brought to the fore. I do not know to what degree this website is accessed by actual sperm donors, but here the connection between producing semen and the sex industry is made explicit, focusing both on the more traditional representation of women as the focal point of erotic labor and on new forms of fantasy where the process of sperm donation itself is eroticized.

CONCLUSION

From the sperm bank perspective, there are different criteria for determining who makes a "good donor." From the clinical perspective, a good donor is someone who is healthy and has abundant, strong-swimming sperm that survives the freezing and thawing process and can successfully fertilize an egg. Socially, a "good donor" is someone who acts appropriately during the sperm donation process, is reliable and easy to work with, and, as one sperm bank worker told me, a good donor is also a guy you "have a good rapport with, someone who is responsible, tall, and honest." A good donor is also someone whose social, educational, and physical characteristics will make him popular among recipients—someone whose sperm will sell. In addition, donor sexuality bridges both clinical and social criteria. Whether explicit or implicit, donor sexuality—including how often a man has sex to ejaculation as well as what kind of sex he engages in—influences the quality and safety of his sperm and semen.

Donor sexuality is both present and absent in the sperm bank industry. It is managed and confined to specific locations, to a point. While sexuality and reproduction appear to be separated by technology, there are still linkages. With sperm donation, a sexual act is inherent to the process, yet there is a glaring absence of references to sex or masturbation in the discourse of most sperm banks, except Rainbow Flag, where male sexuality was assumed and fostered.

Sexuality exists on several levels in the industry. First, it is addressed in relation to the issue of sexual orientation and official policies prohibiting semen donations from gay men. These policies are directly connected to the idea that semen can transmit traits that are "undesirable" and that homosexuality is one of those traits. The rationale behind such policies is that semen can also transmit HIV, though there are medical screening procedures that can reduce this possibility. Second, donor sexuality can cause a potential donor to be screened out (or in), whether it is because of his sexual orientation or the amount or type of sex the donor engages in.

Screening on the basis of sexuality is connected to both official policies surrounding semen donation and the concern with keeping the donor pool medically "safe." A third level of sexuality exists in how sperm banks regulate donor sexual activity and how donors regulate themselves in relation to their work. In fact, some men decide to become sperm donors *because* of their sexuality, thinking that because they are gay, this might be the only way to have a child. Throughout this chapter we have seen a new understanding of sex as an act that is procreative yet solitary.

At TSBC, like most other banks, donation takes place on-site in a very clinical, professional setting. Donor sexuality is ideally contained within the repository. At TSBC the lack of materials or even discourse pertaining to sexuality effectively makes masturbation a clinical—rather than a sexual—process. Here, sexuality (specifically masturbation to climax) is solely for the purpose of procreation. Men who engage in sexual activity to orgasm outside the repository would not be considered to be good donors because the supply of their sperm would be compromised and the safety and quality reduced due to potentially risky sexual practices.

At RFHS, however, donor sexuality outside of donation was assumed but managed. Its donors, though a much higher-risk population, were screened on their sexual practices. A wrong answer—assuming men told the truth about their sexual behaviors—would disqualify a donor. This policy assumed that men would not remain abstinent and attempted to implement controls that would minimize the risk of exposure to HIV and other sexually transmitted diseases.

In an industry where sexuality is at the forefront, it is disguised, contained, and often denied, while altruism—a trait that is incidental to the actual process of sperm donation—is highlighted. The emphasis on altruism is an attempt to erase the sexual and commercial aspects of the sale of sperm and replace them with the more emotionally meaningful notion of sperm (and the resulting child) as a priceless gift and the work as charitable. This framing of a donor's motivations makes them more appealing to women who are looking for sperm donors to create their families. A man who is thought to be in it for the money is usually less desirable than someone who wants to help others create families. Women choosing donors want to be able to tell their future offspring good things about the biological father, and if that child should someday meet him, they want their kid to think he chose to do something nice for a stranger.

5 · GRASSROOTS EUGENICS AND THE FANTASY DONOR

> I've sort of developed this attachment to my donor. He's in the same line of work as me; he looks a lot like me, and he's identity release. And I keep having this fantasy that he and I are standing together at our kid's college graduation, and we're all together having this great time. I hope this donor takes. I think we'd be a great blend.
>
> —Carolyn

> The fairytale father is more grand, more chivalrous, more handsome, more protective, more successful than anyone could ever live up to. Do we really want to compete with a fantasy parent?
>
> —Karleen Pendleton Jimenez (2011, 12)

Choosing a sperm donor is a complicated process. The first consideration is whether to use a known donor or an anonymous sperm bank donor. If a sperm bank donor, then is it better to use a donor who agrees to have his identity released in the future, or one who wishes to remain completely anonymous? Beyond the considerations of a child's having access to his or her genetic origins, women think about what kind of traits they want to see in their future children and what kind of person they are drawn to. Do couples want to match the physical characteristics of the partner who is not carrying the child? Are they drawn to artists or medical students? Do they prefer blond hair and blue eyes or brown hair and eyes? And so on.

In addition to determining the physical traits one prefers, finding the right donor means engaging in a process of defining one's own values and biases. In this chapter, I focus on how women think about the biological, and to some degree social, contributions of the donor to their future child, and how women who use sperm bank donors construct donor identities based on available donor profiles. My main emphasis is on the underlying meanings of donor selection, specifically pertaining to real and imagined men, children, families, and relationships. These fantasies shed light on how people think about genetics and about the sperm cell as the transmitter of genetic information to future offspring. With donor selection, the genetic and the social become conflated.

Cultural and individual notions of "genetic fitness" inform how sperm banks recruit and screen potential donors. These are businesses, with specific clientele, and they need to provide a pool of donors that will be attractive to that clientele. Donors who do not possess characteristics in high demand will produce an unmovable product that takes up precious space in cryogenic tanks. Parallel to the sperm-banking industry, women who screen and select donors participate in a particular form of self-planning—based on cultural assumptions that biology either determines or influences destiny.

When choosing a partner, people think about what kind of person they want to bring into their family and to whom they are attracted. In heterosexual reproductive couplings, a person may overlook aspects they do not necessarily like or find attractive in their partner because love can overwhelm decision making. But in the quest for the "perfect donor," love does not enter into the equation; instead, a kind of pragmatic decision-making process—coupled with individualized perceptions of genetics—comes to the fore. Choosing a donor with specific characteristics is an attempt to stack the deck in favor of creating a child with particular traits. This is what I call grassroots eugenics. Donor selection plays into individual, variable, and imprecise notions of what is genetically valuable. Unlike more formalized positive eugenic programs, like those advocated at the Repository for Germinal Choice, grassroots eugenics has a more liberal twist in that it arises from the stance that women have the right to control their own reproductive choices, to have children (or not) on their own terms—to *choose* their families in very specific ways, through donor selection. Grassroots eugenics turns traditional eugenics on its head; what is considered valuable according to mainstream American standards may or may not be valuable in these alternative arrangements. Race and ancestry, class, gender, and sexual orientation are prioritized in different ways and may challenge social norms. But at the same time, the valuation of some characteristics—like height or education—conforms to mainstream perspectives.

Some of the social anxieties surrounding sperm donation and donor-conceived families have been represented in the mainstream film industry. In the 1990s and early 2000s, sperm donation had not yet become normalized enough for it to be a topic of entertainment. But between 2007 and 2013, titles like *And Then Came Love* (2007), *The Switch* (2010), *The Kids Are All Right* (2010), *The Baby Makers* (2012), and *Delivery Man* (2013) all hit the screen—and usually offered comedic relief for what had once been more controversial. *And Then Came Love* is a film about how a woman eventually falls in love with her anonymous sperm donor when she meets him six years after giving birth to her child. Films such as this echo the dream of the fantasy donor and potential relationship that many straight women have relayed when discussing their sperm donors. *The Kids Are All Right* is about how a lesbian couple of twenty years and their donor-conceived children meet the donor and invite him over to dinner; predictably, one of the women enters into a sexual relationship with him. In the meantime, her partner feels the donor has undermined her authority and her role in her family. When it comes to lesbian sexuality, this film plays into heteronormative fantasies and, at first, prioritizes biological relatedness over social parenthood.

DONOR CHOICE AND GRASSROOTS EUGENICS

Women who undergo donor insemination typically have a variety of traits they seek in a donor. In *Buying Dad,* Harlyn Aizley (2003), a Jewish lesbian living with her partner in Boston, reveals the challenges they faced in the quest for "the perfect donor." Whether using a known donor or an anonymous sperm bank donor, the process of choosing precisely who is complex. Women who decided to use known donors explained that their decision was based on the desire to have a sense of the personality of the person who was going to be the biological father of their child—to like him, to see what he looks like, what kind of person he is. They said using a known donor would help to ensure their child would not grow up with "father fantasies" because he would at least have some contact with them. For example, Anna and Joanne, introduced in chapter 3, both wanted to use a known donor. Joanne explained that her father was absent when she was a child and how that influenced their decision: "I feel really strongly that I want a kid to feel that they have the option of knowing who their father is and physically meeting that person—and not grow up with a sense of wondering. It stems from my experience, obviously, that my father wasn't around and I wasn't able to find him until I was in my twenties. . . . I mean, I grew up with a really close extended family, and my grandfather was always totally there for me. But I still always had these fantasies about my father and what he was like. . . . I don't really want a kid to have to go through that."

Joanne felt there was more to be gained from having a known donor than there were risks. By having a known donor, she could eliminate the risk that her child would grow up reliving her experience of having an absent, "fantasy" father. For her, it was better to know the reality of the person—good or bad—than to grow up imagining what that person might be like and possibly never knowing.

Women who decided to use donors from sperm banks worried that using a known donor would be too risky. The donor might want more of a relationship with the child than they were comfortable with, and might assert paternal rights. At many sperm banks, clients were provided with brief profiles of donors in the pool. These profiles had basic descriptions, including age, height, hair color, education, and profession. Interestingly, sperm donor profiles had far less information than egg donor profiles at clinics and agencies offering egg donations. Most egg donation programs compiled binders of women, categorized according to hair color and ancestry, and included information about the donor's childhood and photographs. I never saw a sperm bank provide donor photographs; however, some sperm bank staff would offer clients some informal indication as to whether they thought the donor was attractive or whether they liked him as a person.

After perusing the one-page basic profile, clients could then narrow down their selection to the top three donor candidates. In some banks, once they had a short list, they could get more detailed profiles, which, at a few sperm banks, were written in the donors' own handwriting. Donor handwriting had elevated significance, as it could give a woman some indication of the donor's personality type. For example, Sharon, Bonnie's partner, explained the significance of their donor's handwritten profile:

> It's funny. You look for these little clues to tell you what kind of person he is. For example, when he filled out the forms there was a place where you're supposed to answer some health history questions and check the boxes if they're in your background or not. And you know, some people are really meticulous and would check every box individually, and some people are more impatient and just draw a line through all of the boxes right down the page. And I'm that kind of impatient person when it comes to filling out forms. Well, this donor drew a line through all of the boxes, and I thought, "Cool! This guy's just like me." I felt like I could relate to this donor.

Sharon—like almost every other woman I talked to—wanted to feel some sort of connection to the donor, whether through looks, handwriting, ancestry, hobbies, common books read, profession, and so on. Women wanted to know that the donor would somehow fit with them or their partner, that they would have common interests and like each other. Thus, something as ordinary as how a person fills out a medical form takes on greater meaning when the real person is a complete mystery.

The one-to-ten-page donor profiles had a great deal of significance for women who chose the biological contributor for their offspring. Women constructed fantasy identities or personalities for donors from their profiles, where the actual identity of the donor is concealed. Women's imagined familiarity with the man behind the genetic material also translated to how they imagined the children who might be born from his donation.

Women fantasize about the donors they chose. They construct identities and personalities out of ten-page profiles. Definitions of family and kinship, distinctions between paternity and fatherhood, the rise of multiple forms of parenthood, and reproductive and nonreproductive relationships all take on new meanings in an ever-changing social world. Creating families through donated (or sold) genetic material gives insight into "the practices of life" and how new social relationships and the production of identity are based on genetic or biological conditions—what Paul Rabinow refers to as "biosociality" (1996).

The perception of genetic material, and the fact that some donors are considered more popular or valuable than others, does have eugenic overtones. But unlike the eugenics movement of the 1930s, and other, more organized and institutionalized applications of eugenic principles, grassroots eugenics is highly variable, depending on one's personal values and preferences regarding what kinds of individuals and families one desires to create. However, grassroots eugenics is still strongly influenced by the notion that desirable and undesirable social and physical traits can be passed down genetically, and that one should give one's potential offspring the best chances possible in life by choosing the right donor. For example, Bonnie described some of the preferences that she and her partner, Sharon, had:

> We wanted someone bright. I wanted someone tall. I think it's an advantage in life. All of them have to be healthy so that sort of goes without saying, but after health came brightness. But, there were certain professions that we thought were smarter than others. Some people seemed too nerdy, you know they played badminton or didn't drink coffee or something. From the information you get on the piece of paper [the donor profile] you just think the doctor who plays basketball and drinks two cups of coffee a day sounds more like our type than the bookkeeper who doesn't drink coffee and plays badminton. . . . The donor we finally picked was a doctor, six foot four, played basketball and drank coffee. We felt like if we met him, we could relate to him, and maybe our child would inherit some of his qualities that we liked.

Ancestry, intelligence, and profession are common concerns when screening donors. Even though the individual or couple is not having a social relationship with the donor, they will have a relationship with any offspring they have through the donor. For women thinking about having children, part of that process is envisioning the type of child one is going to have in one's life. This couple could not envision themselves with a potentially nerdy child who grew up to become a bookkeeper, played badminton, and abstained from coffee—a child they could not relate to. People do not wish to have a child who is not their type, any more than one would want to have a partner who is not one's type. Thus, when people envision their children and their families, they envision having people around them that are like them. Furthermore, since many donors agree to have their identity released to the child, women want men they think their children will be able to meet in the distant future and like.

Another element to grassroots eugenics is a "just in case" interpretation of genetic inheritance. Sandy told me how she screened out a particular donor: "There was one guy who had a really high sperm count and he was Mexican, which I thought about because my daughter's dad is Mexican . . . but I read his narrative and he liked to collect guns and drive cars and I'm like 'No, I don't think so.' I just don't need a little member of the NRA running around. So I'm thinking these things aren't genetically linked, of course they're not. But, I'm thinking to myself, 'Well to some extent, why play with it?'"

Sandy acknowledged the desire for her donor offspring to have a similar ethnic background to her existing child, but was dissuaded from using this donor because she found his hobbies unappealing. She also imagined the potential for her offspring of donor sperm to grow up to be like the donor father. The benefit of having two children with similar ancestral backgrounds was overshadowed by the donor's propensity for collecting guns and driving cars. This was someone Sandy could not imagine herself relating to on a meaningful level nor something she wanted to reproduce.

Although all of the women I spoke to conceded that a child's social environment is just as important as his or her genetic background, they all said that they wanted to give their children the "best chances possible" genetically, "just in case." I heard repeatedly that choosing a donor with a lot of education was a "just in case" scenario, an attempt to stack the deck in favor of a prospective child's lifelong success. Hence one way in which ordinary people attempt to shape their own destiny—and that of their children—is by selecting donors who carry the qualities they desire. For example, Sandy told me how she finally chose the donor with whom she has conceived:

> The amount of education was the first thing I looked for, and then second I looked for whether he had the traits I found attractive. You know, would he look enough like me to be a good blend with the rest of my family, yet not have some of my less desirable qualities like being too fair, or being short and overweight. You think why not stack the deck? I think that's interesting because people meet and marry and/ or have kids for all kinds of reasons and it's not usually is he intelligent enough, is he good looking enough, and yet, in the classic sense of marriage, it is.
>
> It used to be that you marry someone who is from your social class, probably is your religion, and who shares a lot of your values and that's still the norm for marriages and certainly for the ideal marriage. Yet, everybody is out perverting the system at the sperm bank and yet to some extent those values still play in. Do you go for the most different guy you can find or do you go for the guy who seems to be sharing some of my values? And I decided to use someone who seemed to share my values, especially since I was feeling that what I was doing was already a little bit strange.

Although Sandy said having a child through donor insemination is "perverting the system" of the institutions of marriage and family, she made the connection between choosing a donor and choosing a husband—looking for a man to whom you are attracted, who shares your values and education, who seems to be of a similar social class and religious background. She emphasized the importance of finding a donor who seemed familiar in the context of a process that, to her, seemed "a little bit strange." This tendency to seek familiarity when choosing a donor was present among most of the single women I interviewed.

Lesbian couples, too, sought donors who were like them socially. But when choosing a donor, most tried to find men who shared some physical characteristics of the partner who was not attempting to get pregnant at that time. Regina and Nicole, co-mothers of a two-year-old daughter, told me,

> We wanted someone with dark hair, because Regina has dark hair and I have light hair. We wanted a child to look like a blend of the two of us; partially, because we didn't want Regina to have to go out in public alone with the baby and have everyone speculating about their relationship, or saying "Oh, your daughter must look just like your husband." It's funny, though, despite our planning we ended up with a redhead who doesn't look like either one of us, but does look a lot like Regina's brother.

Lesbian couples tended to choose donors in a similar way to how straight couples choose donors—to find someone who looked like their partner. For lesbian couples, though, this can also help lessen the frequency with which one has to "come out," or disclose one's sexual orientation, family structure, and methods of conception, to strangers. For heterosexual couples, choosing a donor who looks like the male partner reduces the chance they will have to "come out" about using a sperm donor at all—especially given that many straight couples even still do not tell anyone when a child is donor-conceived. Both single women and lesbian couples with children frequently fielded questions surrounding whether the child looked like his or her dad. Some women saw these occasions as opportunities to help inform others about different family forms. Other women felt these inquiries were intrusions into their personal lives and responded with short, vague answers designed to put an end to the line of questioning. Either way, women usually chose donors who either most resembled themselves or their partner.

A woman's choice of sperm donors is highly individualistic and influenced by her personal values concerning what type of individual she is attracted to and what kind of relationship possibilities she would like her child to have with the donor; however, there were some common recurrent themes in my interviews. The criteria for donor choice included the degree to which the donor is willing to be known or have his identity disclosed, his ancestry, his intelligence, his body type, his sexual orientation, his hobbies, measures of success (e.g., career and education), and desired physical traits. These personal values are also inseparable from the cultural context in which these women were raised. Choosing a donor, regardless of a woman's relationship status or sexual orientation, has many parallels to choosing a partner or mate. And from early on, individuals learn what kinds of mates are and are not ideal.

ROMANCING THE SPERM

The ways in which donors are recruited and screened in the industry reflects sociogenetic values. Donna Haraway's discussion of "gene fetishism" in the scientific community demonstrates that "the gene is objectified when it seems to be itself the source of value, and those kinds of fetish-objects are the stuff of complex mistakes, denials, and disavowals" (1997, 143). Drawing from Freud, she goes on to state, "Fetishism has to do with a special kind of balancing act between knowledge and belief" (144). The gamete industry selects donors based on their attributes, as well as the knowledge and beliefs surrounding genetics. People purchase gametes according to their own beliefs about heritability and value. Among women attempting to conceive through donor insemination, the gene— as an object of fetish—becomes a reality, a baby, not simply an object of fantasy. Women fantasize about the kind of child they are going to have based, in part, on who they choose as a donor. Semen, as a fetishized commodity, is transformed through the body of the consumer into something else: a child; the desired object has the potential to become a reality that transforms a woman's status from nonmother to mother. At the same time, having to buy sperm to have a child is not most people's first choice. Many experience grief at either not having found a partner to have a child with or not being able to procreate with the partner they have.

Social relations may be disguised through the buying and selling of commodities, but in the case of human gametes (and, I would argue, unlike other body parts, tissues, and fluids that are not generative), social relations become more convoluted, and they also become the stuff of which fantasies are made. For example, as discussed in chapter 3, one woman in my study and her female partner used a known donor. The donor had signed a contract giving away his parental rights but agreed to have some involvement in the child's life. The biological mother's female partner is considered to be the co-parent of the child, and the biological father, or donor, has been given the status of honorary uncle. In this example, biological relations are disguised in order to allow for alternative social relations, where two women and their child compose the primary family unit.

These perceptions of heritability are also connected to perceptions of romance. As Sandy put it, "[Choosing a donor] is like choosing a boyfriend you're never going to meet: you're banking on what kind of person you'd be interested in." Sandy further compared choosing a donor to playing "the dating game": "The donor I finally chose did environmental engineering and sounded very outdoorsy and liked to hike. So, it's kind of like the dating game in that respect. This was somebody who if I met this person I would respect them. I respected the work he did; I respected his views on things. And I think he said basically anyone who wants a child should be able to make a family. And I just thought, well, OK. Anyway, it's a funny process. I mean, you're going through trying to somehow pick up some subtle clue that will tell you this is the right person."

Carolyn also fantasized about her donor and their potential for a future relationship, even though she had not yet conceived. She had gone through ten insemination procedures within the span of a year and had still not gotten pregnant. Despite the numerous failed attempts, she still wanted to continue using the same donor, though another donor may have had a better sperm count or sperm motility. She had fertility issues of her own, but to her knowledge her donor had not yet conceived any children with any other recipients, either. Some women struggle with having to change donors because they become attached to them. As she stated, "I've sort of developed this attachment to my donor. . . . I keep having this fantasy . . ."

The fact that her donor agreed to identity release made her fantasies seem more plausible. Although she had not yet conceived, she talked about having a picture in her head of what the donor looked like and how they would connect with each other because they read the same books, had similar careers, and shared many interests. She romanticized a relationship in her head with a donor she had never met and with a child she had not conceived. In this instance the donor and the child are both in the realm of fantasy and fetish.

These romanticized perceptions of fantasy donors would seem to be more prevalent among single, heterosexual women, but lesbian couples also spoke of choosing a donor as being parallel to dating. For example, Anna and Joanne were seeking a known donor and asked their lesbian friends to think of men who might be suitable:

ANNA: It's a strange phenomenon. We were at this party with mostly lesbian Asian and Latina women and we were asking everyone to help us strategize to find a donor. We told everyone the criteria we were looking for—Latino or Filipino, someone who's cute, reasonably clever, and responsible—and we could overhear everyone talking about it. Someone would make a suggestion and then someone else would say, "No, he's too short," or, "He's not cute enough." And we were thinking, "Well, short doesn't matter," or, "Let us decide if he's cute enough." It was really weird. I felt like I was sixteen years old and a bunch of adolescent girls were drooling over the high school football player. It just seemed weird seeing all these lesbians sitting around talking about men and who they thought was cute. Whoa.

DIANE: So it's kind of like the single matchmaking thing?

JOANNE: Exactly! And there is something very traditional about this whole process too. We had one guy come over who's a friend of a good friend of ours. We made him brunch and we thought he was perfect. It was very traditional making this meal for this man who was coming over to see if he would be a good match for us. This was very strange—modern courting.

This parallel to dating is noted by many women using donor sperm, regardless of the sexual orientation of the recipient or the level of the donor's physical presence in the recipient's life. Yet identity-release donors leave the possibility open that the mother and the donor may eventually meet through the child, leaving fertile ground for ripening fantasies surrounding donor identity—for both the mother and potential offspring.

In some cases, though, choosing a donor can actually lead to new relationships, blurring the distinctions between donor and father, or even in favor of new categories like "duncle" (donor-uncle). Deena, a single, bisexual woman, was thirty-four and in a relationship with Amanda when she first started thinking seriously about having a child.

I really wanted to have kids, and Amanda didn't. And she kept telling me I was wasting my time with her. So she broke up with me. So I was on the phone with Babak—he's a single gay man—and I was telling him about my breakup, crying: "I just need a co-mother." He said, "I'll be your co-mother." And I said, "No, you're not qualified." Then I was thinking about the baby thing and called him a week later and we started talking about him becoming my sperm donor.

So Babak flew out, and did all the screening through the sperm bank in Berkeley. And we started doing the inseminations at home in August of '95. But he lived in New York and at the time and I was in California.

We did the inseminations at my house. It took us some time to get in a groove. He would come and stay over at my house and in the evenings I would do the dishes while he went into my bedroom with a jar and then we'd switch places. He would be sleeping in my living room and I would go to bed and do the insemination. Often we'd do two days in a row or every other day. In all, it was only maybe six or seven tries before I got pregnant, with him flying out from New York whenever I was about to ovulate.

One of the things that happened by June of '96, Babak was living here, he decided to move to California. And it was before I was pregnant, but it was really motivated by wanting to be together. Our relationship evolved over that time and he decided he wanted to be more involved.

Deena's relationship with her friend and donor challenges the "donor" category on many levels. He started out as a good friend whose shoulder she could cry on when her relationship broke up. Through many conversations, they became closer and he became her donor. While they were trying to conceive, Babak made the move to California so he could be closer to Deena as a friend and also have more contact with his future biological child. While their son was conceived outside the bounds of a traditional, heterosexual, romantic relationship, their unique relationship provides both the emotional and physical support Deena seeks and offers Babak the opportunity to be involved in his child's life.

"ETHNIC SPERM"

The concept of "ethnicity" in regard to sperm donation and selection is complicated. The notion of sperm as a transmitter of genetic material—that influences things like hair color, eye color, skin color, and other seen and unseen traits—becomes conflated with social categories and perceptions of cultural and ethnic identity, which are not genetic. No particular skin color, ancestral background, religion, or geographic location defines ethnicity, per se. Max Weber maintains that ethnicity is a "social construct" that is so complex it may be best to abandon the concept ([1922] 1968, [1910] 1971). When it comes to gamete donation, ethnicity is reified as to some degree genetic, rather than social, and has an enormous influence on how people select donors. While the donor may identify with some particular ethnic group, sperm itself has no intrinsic ethnicity. Yet both intended mothers and professionals in the sperm banking industry commonly talked about "ethnic sperm," whether about not being able to find it, not having enough of it, or the potential increased income if they had more of it.

Sperm banks that offer "ethnic sperm" may enjoy increased profits by offering a range of donors from diverse ancestral backgrounds in order to meet the demands of a diverse clientele—especially in the San Francisco Bay Area. Part of the concern over donor ethnicity has to do with the desire to find familiarity and sameness in a process that at times seems rather strange. Women typically expressed the concern that a child conceived to a single mother or a lesbian couple through donor insemination is already going to have enough issues about being "different." Most thought it would be too much of a burden to raise a child who was also "ethnically" different from them, and they felt that they would not have the right tools for teaching a child from a different ancestral background how to get along in the world. For example, Rebecca explained,

> Most of the donors I've used have been Anglo, Irish, Scottish . . . that kind of mongrel mix that my family is. There's one donor that I was very intrigued with, and he was Jewish, and had lost grandparents in the Holocaust, and I made a conscious decision not to use him. He's the only person that I have actually made a decision not to use. I don't know. It's an interesting story for me. People react to this sometimes in different ways, and accuse me of being racist. But, I felt like I couldn't, it felt so strongly to me that his childhood has great-grandparents who died in the Holocaust, that this donor's children should have somebody who can share that with them.

Even though I thought this was a great guy, I didn't feel like I could give that to his children. So, it was sort of like I had children with him, already, and I was already feeling like, "Oooh, there's something that I want you to have, that I can't ever give to you, because I don't know anything about that." You know, of course I'd probably be a great parent to those kids, because I'd really want them to have some understanding of where they came from. But, I couldn't ever raise them through it.

Rebecca expressed the idea that parents have the responsibility to pass down cultural knowledge to their children. To have a child who is not of one's ethnicity, and who does not have access to his or her cultural heritage through the second parent, is seen as being irresponsible.

Yet some women, like Deena, see their donor-conceived children as a way of bridging divides: "Babak is Pakistani and Muslim, and I'm Jewish. I really want our son to appreciate his mixed heritage. I think it's pretty neat he's a Jewish and Muslim baby, and I'd like him to know about all of that heritage—especially since he looks somewhat Pakistani. He's my little contribution toward world peace."

Since Deena used a known donor, and her donor is part of her child's life, she did not feel the burden of having to be the only parent to pass down cultural knowledge to her child, as Rebecca did.

Often, the choice to screen out a donor because of ethnicity is based not on any concrete concern about a child's being ethnically different but rather on idiosyncratic biases that are not even fully understood by the people who hold them and are not consistent with what is normally considered to be racist or prejudice. For example, Sharon and Bonnie explained how they ruled out certain donors because of ethnicity: "Sharon has a thing against anyone with a German background, because of all of the atrocities against Jews and gays in World War II. And we both had a thing against people from Ireland—although I'm not sure why. For some reason, you know if you can choose, the guy from Yugoslavia sounds a lot more interesting than the guy whose family is from Ireland."

Although neither of these women is Jewish (but both are lesbians), for Sharon and Bonnie, the decision not to choose a donor with a Germanic background was rooted in a political view that they did not want to produce more people whose ancestors came from a country that committed crimes against humanity. Here, the sperm is perceived as something that has the power to carry and transmit a horrible legacy—at least symbolically. Ironically, this stance is the antithesis of the motivations behind 1930s eugenics but is still rooted in the eugenic notion that the genes of a race are responsible for the actions of certain people.

People do not always recognize their reasoning behind ruling out a particular ethnic group. For example, Bonnie and Sharon did not want a donor with an Irish background. They were not sure why, but it just did not appeal to them. The ways in which ethnicity and identity are thought about and imagined do not always make sense. Most women have notions of what they find appealing or unappealing, and these are not always rooted in logic or politics.

Joanne and Anna, who are Latina and Filipina, respectively, are trying to find a known donor who is Asian, Hispanic, or Latino. Their quest to find a donor that meets their ethnicity criteria has been a difficult task.

ANNA: The whole ethnicity thing has been a real trauma—it's the main sticking point. At the sperm banks, all the donors are white, and even though we're trying to find a known donor it seems like we're still only able to find guys who are white that are willing to do this. . . . And using a known donor, I mean, this process becomes really public. We tell our friends and family about what we're looking for in a donor, and my sister says, "Why are you so stuck on finding someone who is Filipino?" Then it becomes really personal. You have to unravel all your issues about ethnicity and assimilation and race and production, reproduction, culture, and all this stuff, and have to defend yourself. Then people start picking on you because of that.

DIANE: It sounds to me like some of the ideas of what you want in a donor are part of your political stance.

ANNA: Oh, totally. And people don't seem to get it. We have this one friend who is white and he kind of hinted that he wanted to be a donor. And I had to explain to him all these complex reasons why we want someone close to our ethnic mix, about the politics of race, culture and so on, and at the end of it he just looked at me and said, "So, you're basing your decision on picking a donor depending on how that person looks?" And I said, "No, I didn't say that! There are all these complex reasons that come into play." And it's like he didn't even hear me.

Ethnic considerations in selecting semen donors are extremely complex and correspond to women's desire to have a child that is like them, as well as broader political issues surrounding culture, identity, and power in American society. When choosing a donor, women are forced to confront their own issues and biases surrounding ethnicity, intelligence, social class, and so on. For women undergoing donor insemination, choosing a donor is perceived as choosing the kind of child one wishes to bring into one's life.

INFERTILITY AND REDRAWING THE LINES

While, at first, changing donors may feel overwhelming, after a long span of trying unsuccessfully to conceive, for some women, changing donors becomes less significant. The primary goal becomes finding a donor who will get them pregnant. For example, one couple, Heather (thirty-five) and Stephanie (forty-one), have been together for thirteen years. Heather had been trying to conceive for three years, and she discussed how their criteria for choosing a donor changed throughout the process of seeking treatment for infertility:

> At first we were really attached to the idea of using a known donor, or at least an identity-release donor. We had this whole list of, he had to be smart, attractive, and seem like a nice guy. Now, at this point, it's "Give me a high sperm count. Give me the most loaded count you can come up with."
>
> It's weird, at the beginning you have these limits or these criteria of what you want in a donor, what kinds of medical treatment you will and won't do. But the lines just keep getting erased and redrawn, erased and redrawn, erased and redrawn, until you find yourself doing treatments you never thought you would do, and buying sperm of one donor just because the bank has a two-for-one deal on him that week. You think, "Oh good, two vials for the price of one." You think it's more sperm for your money, but it really isn't. They're selling it two-for-one because his count was low that time. But you just do whatever you can to feel like you've increased your chances. Now, I kind of joke about it sometimes, you know? I'm a lesbian but I've had more sperm in me than a prostitute.

Heather's story touches on several important issues. First, it demonstrates how women's criteria for choosing a donor change as they become further entrenched in the world of infertility treatment. Initially, a good donor is considered to be someone who is intelligent, attractive, or identity release. As repeated attempts at conception fail, a good donor is redefined as someone who has a high sperm count. Thus the notion of quality sperm shifts from a more culturally based perception of "quality individuals" to a more concrete, biological reality of quantity and quality of sperm.

This also corresponds to how Heather perceived the "two-for-one deal" offered by the sperm bank. She felt as though she got more for her money since she got double the amount of semen. However, the amount of *sperm* contained within those samples was actually no more than what she would usually get in one vial, since it was a poor sample. The sperm bank, then, offers promotions on products they want to move out of their stock, and the consumer purchases them thinking she is getting a deal.

Second, Heather described how after repeated attempts at conception failed, she found herself redrawing the lines as to what she considered acceptable infertility treatment. Women who experience difficulty conceiving frequently start off with a list of procedures or pharmaceuticals they would never consider. When conception does not occur, they become increasingly desperate and begin to embrace—even search out—treatments they were initially against. Thus experiences of infertility cause women to adapt their personal boundaries in order to increase their chances at reproductive success. This often becomes problematic for a relationship when the woman's partner still holds to the original boundaries regarding medical intervention and tries to encourage her partner to stop treatment, and the woman trying to conceive a child is looking for the next procedure that might offer the possibility of hope.

A final observation regarding Heather's story has to do with how infertility (and donor insemination) affects a woman's perception and experience of her sexuality. Heather, a lesbian, equated the experience of having the semen of numerous different men in her body with being "like a prostitute." In some heterosexual couples using donor insemination, men told me they had this irrational feeling that their wives had cheated on them. On a symbolic level, sexuality and reproduction are intrinsically connected—even when separated by technology and sexual orientation. Technological reproduction does not completely obliterate the perception of sexuality, even when sex is separate from conception.

CONCLUSION

This chapter has explored how donor selection is embedded in cultural assumptions surrounding genetic inheritance. Some donors' genetic contributions are valued over others, in ways that both reflect and challenge prevailing social standards. While, in some ways, single women and lesbian couples having children through donor insemination are—as Sandy put it—"perverting the system," at the same time, there is something very conventional about how women decide to become mothers using donor sperm, how they choose a donor, and how they move forward to create and define their families. Donor choice reflects a person's, or couple's, values, and, in some ways, the process parallels choosing a partner.

Women spend significant time and energy deliberating over how to choose the right donor for their future child. Donor selection forces people to confront their own biases in terms of what characteristics they value and want to see passed down to their children. Most of the time, the lay perceptions of genetics that guide these choices have no basis in the scientific facts of genetic inheritance but rather reflect individuals' (and couples') desires to create a social and moral order that reflects their own personal politics by creating family. I refer to this as "grassroots eugenics"—where the personal and the presumed biological become political.

Romance and fantasy enter the picture—even when the conception process is seemingly detached and clinical and completely separated from reproduction. Some women think about future possibilities with their donors. Women using known donors or friends may even build relationships with the donors, who may take on active roles in their children's lives and become more like fathers—though categorized as "uncles" and "friends"—than some children's legally defined fathers. Family structure is reimagined to fit new circumstances, made possible by technology and a changing society.

6 · SEMEN AS GIFT, SEMEN AS GOODS

Reproductive Workers and the Market in Altruism

I started thinking about it in college when a friend told me he was doing this donor gig and getting paid thirty-five bucks a time. I said, "Wow!" I figured if you want to satisfy yourself and you want to help other people, why not get paid to do it?   —Jake, twenty-five, anonymous sperm bank donor

The couple hundred dollars I made wasn't what motivated me. You have to go through all these blood tests, drive back and forth, and go through a whole screening before you ever get selected. It wasn't even enough to pay for my time.   —Robert, thirty-three, donor at Rainbow Flag Health Services

Sperm donation is simultaneously conceptualized as gift and product, exposing a tension between monetary and altruistic donor motivations. Aside from providing basic descriptive, genetic, education, and family history information, donors fill out donor narratives. These narratives can include questions such as, "What are your hobbies and interests?" "What are your life's ambitions?" "What would you like to tell the recipients of your sperm?" "What would you like to tell the children born from your sperm?" "Why do you want to become a sperm donor?" and so on. When donors write their profiles, sometimes sperm bank staff offer guidance on what to write that will make them more appealing to potential recipients. In addition to his other characteristics, how a donor frames his motivations can affect his appeal to potential recipients.

The questions vary somewhat from one sperm bank to the next, but these profiles give intended parents a sense of the person providing genetic material for their child. Most parents keep these profiles and plan to share them with their children eventually. When sorting through the profiles, clients are looking for donors who speak to them, who make them feel a connection in some way. If a

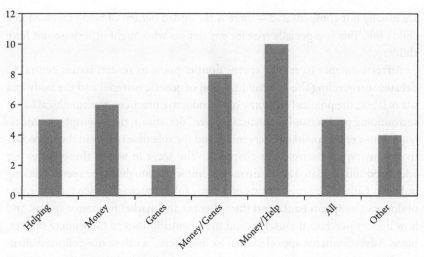

FIGURE 6.1 Sperm donor motivations.
SOURCE: Donor profiles from TSBC (*n* = 33).

donor answers the "Why do you want to be a donor" question with, "For the money," he is not going to be as desirable as someone who says, "Because my sister just had a child with donor sperm. I see what that gift did for our family, so I wanted to pass that on to someone else."

To explore the question of donor motivation, in addition to my interviews, I analyzed thirty-three donor profiles from one sperm bank in 1995. Their responses could be broken down into three main categories: helping others, earning money, passing down genes, any combination of the three, and other responses, as seen in figure 6.1.

Responses were close to equally divided between men who were donating solely to help someone else and men who were solely providing sperm for money. Ten donors expressed a combined motivation of money and a desire to help other people have children, and eight responses focused on a combination of money and passing on their genes. One donor gave a rather flippant response, stating that sperm donation offered "great hours, good pay, good benefits, and a week in the Mediterranean." Another fell mostly into the money category but wanted to put what he made toward his brother's education. And another, who had a one-year-old brother conceived via donor egg, fell mostly into the helping category. Several of the respondents who selected genetic reasons also stated that they did not see having kids in the future themselves, and one stated that his wife was infertile so he wanted to help someone else. Although this is not a huge sample, it does point to the fact that men's motivations to become a sperm donor are complex, merging multiple motivations simultaneously, including earning money, helping others, and passing on their genetic material. In the case of known donors—who are usually not compensated—there is the added benefit of being involved in a child's life. This is especially true for gay donors who might otherwise not have children.

Advertisements to recruit sperm donors point to several issues central to debates surrounding the commodification of genetic material and the body as a site of labor: the political economy of reproductive practices, the bioethical issues surrounding paid versus "altruistically given" donations, the assumptions underlying donor recruitment and screening, and the role of sexuality in the reproductive industry, as discussed in chapter 4. The ways in which these issues are addressed and regulated are by no means uniform throughout the sperm-banking industry. Cultural interpretations of genetic inheritance influence the screening of donors (by sperm banks and their clients), the market for donor sperm, and how donors perceive themselves and their contributions to the gamete marketplace. Advertisements appeal to men to "be a hero," a call to masculinized altruism. For prospective egg donors, the messaging is slightly different; "be an angel" is the feminized altruistic recruitment message. The message to make money while helping others is found in both egg and sperm donor advertisements.

Throughout the sperm-banking industry, as well as among consumers who purchase semen for reproduction, certain donor characteristics are thought to be of higher value than others. Good physical health is of primary importance; without it, one would not normally pass screening procedures for becoming a donor. Beyond that, the perceived value of a donor becomes more complex: physical traits like height, weight, and hair and eye color; social traits like education, "personality," motivation for becoming a donor, and willingness to be identified; and more blurry traits like ethnicity and intelligence have varying values depending on both the repository doing the screening and consumer demands. The ultimate question here is, How do locally held perceptions of what semen is thought to contain affect its exchange value?

The perceived "quality" of semen as both commodity and genetic material is strongly connected to the replication of a variety of U.S. cultural ideals, including an emphasis on altruism, intelligence, and other characteristics that are perceived to be transmittable by the sperm itself. Many sperm bank employees, as well as recipients, typically discuss donor sperm as if it had a personality of its own that would be exhibited by the offspring of that sperm, regardless of the biological contributions of the mother or the environmental conditions in which the offspring was to be raised.

Numerous parallels can be drawn between semen donation and the entire industry in body parts—organs, blood, gametes, and so on—especially in regard to the comparative value assigned to that which is donated, as opposed to that which is sold, as well as the perceptions of what makes a "good" donor. Medical anthropologists conducting research on organ donation, for example, have pointed out the importance of anonymous altruism among organ donors for recipients and their families, acknowledging the organ as the "gift of life" (Sharp 1995) and identifying the "tyranny of the gift" for living donors in the global black market in human organs (Scheper-Hughes 2000, 2007).This rhetoric of gift and altruism is rife within the sperm-banking industry as well, and it affects the selection and screening of donors by both sperm banks and recipients. Similar euphemisms of semen as the "gift of life" abound among clients who have borne children of donor sperm.

Rene Almeling (2011, 2017) argues that in the gamete industry, sperm dona-tion is framed as a job and egg donation as a gift, due to a gendered division of labor and different sets of assumptions surrounding male and female perceptions of the children conceived through their donations. In turn, she argues that the rhe-toric used in donation programs "shapes how donors understand the exchange of sex cells for money" (2017, 6). This is true to a degree—the language used in sperm banks and egg donation programs does influence how gamete donors inter-pret and talk about what donation means, and sometimes this includes a gen-dered framework. However, while there certainly are gendered aspects to sperm and egg donation, my results indicate that the "job = masculine" and "gift = feminine" argument does not sufficiently address the complexity of the issue— both in the framing on the industry's side and in how sperm and egg donors think about their donations. Professionals who work in sperm banks and egg donation programs both refer to the financial benefits for "donors," as well as the benefit of helping someone have a child; both refer to "donation" as simultaneously a "job" and "not a job," as compensation is framed as merely "reimbursement for time and trouble" for providing an enormous "gift." Likewise, sperm donors perceive their donations as gifts *and* work *and* have a genetic interest as well.

In my current research in which I have interviewed over ninety egg donors and an array of professionals in the industry, I have discovered egg donors' motiva-tions are also mixed and complex. Egg donation industry professionals frame the meanings of gametes and gamete donation/sale in variable ways. Instead of the dichotomy of "job" versus "gift," what I see is a collage of motivations and per-ceptions for both sperm and egg providers, with some people more motivated by money, others more motivated by helping others, and others uncertain whether they will have children of their own and wanting to ensure their genetic continuation—regardless of gender. Sperm banks and egg agencies also play a role in framing what donations mean, to both their donors and the intended parents. Furthermore, the concepts of "gift" and "job" are held simultaneously in both of these gamete donation spaces. Both male and female gamete providers sometimes talk about "donating" for a "paycheck" that helps them make ends meet while simultaneously helping others create families. The fact that egg donors are now taxed by the Internal Revenue Service on their income from their "donations" as independent contractors—and sperm donors are not—even further reveals the complexities of how to categorize reproductive work, both within and outside the industry.

So how does gender play out in the gamete industry? For one, the amount of visual information available on sperm donors and egg donors varies dramatically. Women who provide eggs usually submit an array of photographs of their family, themselves as children, and sometimes even themselves as adults, and these photographs are posted in online donor profiles. It is also not uncommon for egg donor programs to provide videos of their donors. In the early 1990s, before profiles were made available online, egg donor profiles were housed in binders, categorized by hair color and ancestry, and included an array of photographs. Rarely have I seen online profiles with sperm donors' photos, and I only know of one clinic where intended parents could get a video of their sperm donor to give to their child at some point in the future. While a sperm bank worker may give hints that a certain donor is particularly attractive, the clients will not have access to any visual material.

The difference in the visual representation of sperm and egg providers is partially due to how intended parents select donors: they want egg donors who are pretty first and smart second, and sperm donors who are smart, successful, and tall first, with handsome a close second. These visual representations—or lack thereof—resonate with how women and men are differentially depicted in media, fashion magazines, and popular culture. Jennifer Siebel Newsom's Representation Project, and her film *Miss Representation*, addresses how the media sells the idea that "girls' and women's value lies in their youth, beauty, and sexuality" (http://therepresentationproject.org/film/miss-representation/). The representation of donors in the gamete industry very much reflects these gendered stereotypes. The industry readily highlights an egg donor's beauty. But a sperm donor's attractiveness is considered far less important than his intellectual capabilities—despite the lack of evidence that only males contribute intelligence to future offspring.

The cultural significance of semen, as a source of genetic material, and what it is thought to contain, affects its value as a commercial product. Sperm is reified as something that contains a personality, an ethnicity, and a risk. The cultural values of altruism attempt to decommodify the commodity—to remove semen's status as a marketable product and redefine it as gift. In the sperm-banking industry, how gift language is used varies, depending on the overall mission of a particular sperm bank. The Repository for Germinal Choice (RGC), for example, framed its business and promotional materials to highlight altruism and "giving children the best possible start" while "improving the human gene pool." Rainbow Flag Health Services (RFHS) sought to build the LGBTQ community through donor insemination and also highlighted donor altruism. The Sperm Bank of California (TSBC) has a more business-minded approach and recognizes donors' need for money while providing the "gift." Other gamete businesses, like California Cryobank—where I did not conduct fieldwork—are located even further on the business end of spectrum but still blend monetary and altruistic incentives in their recruitment advertisements for both sperm and egg donors. Each sperm bank can be thought of as having its own cultural environment, which is influenced by its particular business model and underlying philosophies regarding the perception of donations as commodities or gifts, as well as the question of donation being a "job" or "altruistically motivated." For most, it is mixture of both, but on a spectrum.

COMMODITIES, GIFTS, AND SEMINAL VALUE

> The producer who carries on exchange feels ... that he is exchanging more than a product of hours of working time, but that he is giving something of himself—his time, his life. Thus he wishes to be rewarded, even if only moderately, for this gift. To refuse him this reward is to make him become idle or less productive.   —Marcel Mauss (1954, 77)

> A commodity is, in the first place, an object outside us, a thing that by its properties satisfies human wants of some sort or another. The nature of such wants, whether, for instance, they spring from the stomach or from fancy, makes no difference.   —Karl Marx (1906, 41)

Throughout the anthropological literature, the concept of the gift is discussed in terms of how social relations are formed and solidified through the act of gift giving. Drawing on Marcel Mauss (1954), the gift itself is not considered important; what is significant is the system of complex social relations one enters into through the acts of giving and receiving. Furthermore, gifts are typically distinguished from commodities, items that are bought and sold, as in the latter, social relations between persons are disguised behind the transfer of money and goods. Arjun Appadurai (1986) has critiqued the simplification of distinctions between gifts and commodities in much of the anthropological writing on the subject, and he has argued (along with Bourdieu 1977) that gift exchange is a particular form of the circulation of commodities.

Transactions involving the giving, buying, and selling of semen further blur the distinctions between gift and commodity exchanges. Semen, as a product that is bought and sold, marketed, categorized, screened, and so on, appears to be a commodity. It appears that the person purchasing the semen in order to conceive a child pays her money, takes her product home, and hopefully gets the desired result—a pregnancy and a child. These transactions, however, though attempting to deny the social relations of "fatherhood," cannot escape them. First, the donor who provides semen for a woman's child becomes the subject of fantasy and fetish—some sort of social relationship exists, at least in the realm of the imagination and certainly in the realm of the biological, should a child be conceived. The economic and emotional value of the imagined donor varies depending on the traits he is thought to possess. Second, the recipient may, at some point, have some sort of contact with the semen donor, who often has the option of entering into a social relationship with the offspring as the child's biological father, albeit a limited one. Thus there is the possibility for a delayed gift-countergift interaction that is not usually present in the circulation of commodities. Third, the notion of semen as commodity is further confused by the fact that the recipients themselves perceive the donor as having given them a precious "gift" (a child, or even just the potential to have a child), although the women have paid for it. Semen transactions, then, conflate the gift-commodity distinction.

In adoption, these issues are paralleled—and extended; only here, actual children are the commodities rather than the genetic material that can result in a child. Viviana A. Zelizer (1994) analyzes the interactions between market or price and personal and moral values in reference to shifting cultural interpretations of childhood since the Industrial Revolution—a time when the economic value of a child's contribution to the household disappeared, but the emotional value of the child increased. In regard to adoption, and a black market in babies, she discusses a contradiction between a cultural system that "declared children priceless emotional assets, and a social arrangement that treated them as cash commodities" (201). International, public, and transracial adoptions are also embedded in race, class, and gender controversies, in which some children are perceived to have more value than others, and some families are targeted more than others for the adoption market (Gailey 2010). Judith Modell explores how adoption challenges our core symbols of kinship, and she examines the significance of biological and cultural interpretations of kinship (1994) and formations of identity. The social and legal debates surrounding the buying and selling of babies through adoption agencies and independent agents center on conflicting themes of the market's need to meet consumer demands and the moral values that emphasize parenting as a gift that should be motivated by altruism, not profit. The child itself—or the potential to create a child—has an economic value that is based solely on the emotional rewards, not on the child's potential to contribute economically to the family.

In discussing the relative value of commodities in economic exchange, Appadurai argues that politics "creates the link between exchange and value." The value of property or objects is not inherent in the thing itself but rather is determined by the "judgment made about them by subjects." He further argues, "Commodities, like persons, have social lives" (1986, 3). But how is the value of semen as both gift and commodity determined when the product is not only a product but also something that comes from a person and aids in creating other persons who will, themselves, be engaged in social relations, and who may at some point enter into a social relationship with the biological donor who sired them? Furthermore, how is the value of semen connected to the judgments subjects make about what constitutes a quality person? This comes down to the question of the *phenomenology of exchange* that is at play when the commodity that is purchased enters into and becomes part of one's body, and eventually becomes another person with his or her own social history. Marx (1906, 82) notes that commodities are transformed through the process of exchange, and he uses the example that wood is transformed into a table by the person who purchases it. With the exchange of semen this is no less true: with seminal exchange, the gamete can be transformed into a child by the woman who purchases it. The fact that the product is a child, a person, rather than a material object like a table, makes the significance of social relations in commodity exchange more pronounced.

The social relations in seminal exchange are quite complex. Typically, unless a woman is using a known donor, the exchange of semen is between donor and sperm bank, and then sperm bank and recipient. The buyer and the seller of the product are not directly involved in the act of exchange with one another. Despite the physical distance between the seller and the purchaser, semen is often perceived as a very intimate "gift" for the women who have bought it, and the donor is perceived as having given the woman the "gift of life," a child. Women express their unending gratitude for this man whom they have never met because he gave them something they consider precious. Despite the fact that semen transactions are commodity exchanges, women typically perceive this exchange as a type of gifting, and they fantasize about how alliances with the donor could be forged in the future, when the child reaches the age at which a donor's identity may be released. For example, in chapter 5, Carolyn explained how she fantasized that she would get pregnant by her donor and would someday be standing with her imaginary daughter and her imaginary donor together at her imaginary daughter's graduation. Thus the possibility for social interaction through gift exchange both is delayed and is the subject of fantasy and fetishism.

Despite semen's quality as a commodity, there exists a strong motivation to emphasize its value as a purely altruistically given gift among individual women who purchase it, as well as among sperm bank representatives. For women, the altruistic character of the donor is important. It gives them something positive to tell their children about the man who helped to make their lives possible. Being able to tell one's child that his or her donor wanted to help people has given families has much greater emotional value than having to tell the child that the donor needed the money. Hence, when women decide on a donor, they often look for clues in the donor profiles that will tell them that the donor was motivated—at least partially—by a desire to help others. Ironically, a sperm donor who appears to be more altruistically motivated carries greater emotional and economic value than someone who is primarily motivated by money.

DONOR TYPOLOGIES

Sperm donors receive financial remuneration to varying degrees. Some repositories, like RGC, do not pay their donors at all; some, like RFHS, offer very little
and define payment in terms of reimbursing donors for their time and trouble;
and some pay donors between forty and fifty dollars per semen sample. In all of
the sperm banks where I conducted fieldwork—whether donors were paid or
not—the idea of financially compensating a donor for providing semen is not
neutral. Here, I will explore the varying degrees to which semen donors are compensated, as well as how sperm repository representatives interpret the meaning
of exchanging money for human gametes. In this section, I offer donor typolo-
gies, some of which are borrowed from Richard Titmuss's ([1970] 1997) work on
blood donors.

The Paid Sperm Bank Donor

At many sperm banks, donors are paid for their time and their "donations." A paid
sperm bank donor could either be anonymous or unknown but willing to have
his identity released to the child at some point in the future. Paid donors are often
recruited through college newspapers and online advertisements. Advertisements
specifically offer a monetary reward for one aspect of male sexuality that produces
a certain product—semen. Most ads, however, combine financial and altruistic
incentives by appealing to men to "be a hero" and help someone have a child, similar to the "be an angel" appeal of egg donor ads. Donors—whether they are providing sperm or eggs—internalize the messages they receive from advertisements
and through the recruitment and screening process.

Paid donors become part of a market in which their ability to bring themselves
to climax produces a commodity that is bought and sold, thereby linking their
sexuality to the market for genetic material. A further notion, here, is one of waste:
Since a man is already masturbating anyway, why not get paid for it rather than
wasting sperm that could be valuable?

Some in the sperm-banking industry feel that a paid donor has a vested interest in concealing personal information—for example, his health or sexual practices or family history of genetic diseases. Screening of donors is important to
guarantee a lower level of risk for both the recipient and the potential offspring.
Among sperm repositories that pay their donors, it is thought that these screening procedures are enough to ensure the product's safety.

Sperm donors also must regulate their sexual activity. They should abstain from
ejaculating at least two to three days before a sample is collected. If a donor has
too much sexual activity, or ejaculates too close to his scheduled donation, his
sperm count will be too low. As one worker at a sperm bank states, "If a guy is
playing ball [i.e., having sexual intercourse] with his partner usually he wouldn't
make a good donor." In some cases when the count is lower than usual or the

sperm is not of high quality, the repository may pay the donor less than his usual rate and may also offer the recipients two vials for the price of one. This is obviously at some extra cost to the sperm bank.

Jake told me how he regulates his own sexuality—both slowing his quest for companionship and reducing his own solitary sexual activities—so that he can provide a quality sample and receive maximum payment. "If I wasn't a sperm donor I'd be much more interested in having a girlfriend. One time I went to my appointment, but two days before I had watched a porn movie. When I went to the sperm bank and provided a sample, they tested it and they said my count was low, so they paid me half of what I usually got. Kinda pissed me off, but I guess it was my own fault. Now I make sure to reschedule if I end up, you know."

Although paid donors are primarily motivated by the cash reward—approximately fifty dollars per specimen in the 1990s—they typically identified other factors in their decision to become donors as well—for example, wanting to help other people have children, a secondary altruism. The donors who express such "higher reasons" for becoming donors are thought to have more value than those who are just in it for the money. A "good" donor is someone who is committed, who has thought the process through, and who is doing it for altruistic as well as monetary reasons.

Many donors take on a semiprofessional status. That is, they make regular donations (multiple times a month) for usually at least a year. These donors generally enter into a "long-term relationship" with the sperm bank—keeping its staff abreast of things that might affect the quality of their semen. Barbara Raboy, cofounder of TSBC, said she works to gain this kind of trust and commitment from her donors, as well as her clients: "You keep seeing the same donors over and over again. One gentleman, for example, has been with us and he's due for his annual work-up, so he's going to go see our physician for his physical. This is exactly what you want with your donors because you develop this kind of partnership with them over time and you get to know them really well."

This notion of building a partnership or a relationship with the donors was present at all the sperm banks where I conducted interviews. The ability of repository representatives to get to know their donors, to build a relationship with them, and to trust them—to have a commitment from them—is considered extremely important to the smooth operation of the repository. This notion of trust between donors and sperm bank operators is extremely significant for understanding the cohesive social relations surrounding semen exchange. Because semen, as a commodity, also contains potential risk—for example, of passing on sexually transmitted as well as genetic diseases—the ability to trust donors is of utmost importance. Indeed, one sperm bank was recently sued by a recipient couple for providing semen that carried a genetically linked kidney disease that was transmitted to their children.[1]

The Reimbursed Voluntary Donor

At some sperm banks, minimal payment is given to voluntary donors. This form of financial reward is not viewed as payment per se but rather is seen as reimbursement for the donor's time and the "labor" expended by the donor to produce the product, as well as compensation for the inconvenience of the process. As Leland explained,

> When you pay a donor you get into the whole thing about what is the morality about paying someone for their reproductive tissues. Why is that different than paying someone to donate a kidney, for example? Now I do pay my donors but it's a very small amount and it's primarily a stipend for their inconvenience in terms of getting here. It's a maximum of $200 that comes at the end of the program. They come here and they give all these donations and they go through physical exams and have all this blood drawn, they get poked and prodded and six months later they come back and get their blood drawn again and after that then they get their $200. For a lot of them that travel significant distances they're clearly not in it for the money.

For Leland, there was a limit to what a donor could be paid and still not be "in it for the money"—still be a legitimate donor, rather than someone who exploits his own genetic material for financial gain; although, Leland failed to point out that by paying donors less, he was potentially seeing increased profits from the sale of semen. He also mentioned that if a donor is getting paid for his product, he has a vested interest in lying about any diseases he may carry. At this sperm bank, financial compensation of donors was believed to undermine the relationship of trust seen as necessary between donors and sperm banks. Leland also felt that paying donors for their semen is unethical, similar to selling a kidney.

Anonymous versus Open-Identity Donors

At some sperm banks, donors have the option to have their identity released when the offspring reaches a certain age, usually eighteen. Two banks in this research, RFHS and TSBC, both offered donors whose identity could or would be released. At RFHS it was mandatory when the offspring reached three months of age, at which point Leland contacted the mother and provided her with the donor's contact information, then called the donor and told him that a child had been born. At TSBC at the time of my research, it was optional for donors to have their identity released when the child reached eighteen; now it is mandatory. If a donor agrees to have his identity released, he cannot change his mind, however. Many other sperm banks, including RGC, prohibit the release of donor identities and do not offer this as an option.

At most sperm banks that offer them, open-identity donors are in much higher demand than those who wish to remain anonymous. Most recipients want their offspring to at least have the opportunity to seek out their donors should they so choose. Many women also feel that identity-release donors have thought the process through more deeply and have taken greater personal responsibility in regard to the offspring their sperm produces. Donors do not receive more money if they agree to have their identity released. However, at one California sperm bank in the 1990s, open-identity semen did cost approximately twenty-five dollars more per vial than non-identity-release semen because it was in higher demand. In 2002 TSBC did start charging more for identity-release sperm because anonymous sperm was not selling. The value of semen, then, is subject to the laws of supply and demand, and future access to donor identity increases a donor's value.

DONOR ALTRUISM AND SEMINAL VALUE

Sperm bank policies regarding paying donors express conflicting notions of what it "should" mean to be a donor and what the "right reasons" are for donation. At RFHS, Leland felt if a man was a donor "for the money," then he had a vested interest in lying on the intake forms about his health, sexual practices, and other issues. At other banks—for example, TSBC—staff felt that a donor was providing a service, sometimes at great personal sacrifice, and should be financially rewarded. Still, the issue of altruism and trust is an important one. These conceptions of the commercial as bad and the voluntary as good are the topic of Titmuss's treatise on donor blood, and they permeate the sperm-banking industry as well.

In *The Gift Relationship* ([1970] 1997), Titmuss provides a comparative analysis of blood donation in the United States and the United Kingdom, exploring altruism and the gifting of blood in comparison with the marketing and commodification of blood. These arguments are extremely relevant to the discussion of semen donation and the perceived tension between those who give it freely and those who expect reimbursement for their "labor." According to Titmuss, the anonymous gift of blood is the archetype of a pure gift relationship because the donor does not have any motivation for donating other than the desire to help others. However, the question remains whether any gift is driven by pure altruism. For example, the "altruistic" blood donor may feel personal satisfaction that he or she is being a good person by donating blood. Thus, personal satisfaction is the motivation for being a donor, rather than pure altruism. I argue that, in the case of semen donation, there is always some form of self-interest among donors— even when the semen is given freely and the donor remains anonymous.

Blood and semen are parallel fluids in many ways: they are both regenerative; they both can be donated or sold; they are both perceived and experienced as a "gift of life"; they can both be stored in banks before they are received by recipients; they are both potential transmitters of HIV/AIDS and other diseases and are thus subject to numerous testing procedures to ensure safety for their recipients; and they both forge some kind of relationship between the donor and recipient—even though they may never actually meet. Because of their regenerative quality, their donation and sale have not fallen under the same strictures as have the donation and sale of human organs.

In the sperm-banking industry, the identification of altruistically donated semen as good and purchased semen as bad is apparent but not consistently articulated. At TSBC, for example, semen donors are paid, but someone who is donating just for the money is not the ideal. The best donors are considered to be those who also have some personal reason for donating—for example, if the donor had a relative who went through infertility or had a baby through donor insemination, and the donor would like to be able to "give that gift to someone else." Sperm banks realize that most men donate because they are in college and need the money, yet they believe donors should be motivated by more than just monetary compensation. This is often a trait that women look for when they study the donor profiles to select a donor.

Other repositories—for example, RFHS—provide minimal compensation for the donors' "inconvenience," and RGC has a policy against donor compensation. Both these repositories feel that to compensate donors monetarily would give them a vested interest in lying on their applications and thus make them less trustworthy as donors and increase their risk for transmitting genetic or other diseases. As Leland stated,

> Most sperm banks don't have very good controls on their own system because if you're a sperm donor and you're being paid fifty dollars a shot you have a financial interest. So what if your family is rife with diabetes or heart disease. You lie, you say, "I have none of that in my family," and no one is ever going to find out. Well, if my guys lie to me, they're going to meet this woman and if they find out that their child has a genetic disorder, and therefore the donor might too, they have been defrauded and that would probably be actionable. So, actually I have better controls on making sure that my guys are honest than the rest of the industry does.

Similarly, Robert K. Graham, the founder of RGC, stated in a video-recorded interview, "We think it wrong to pay donors. It produces a bad motivation. Our donors realize that they are exceptionally gifted in their hereditary endowment, and that they can share this great gift with youngsters yet to be born without diminishing themselves in any significant way. So they are highly motivated and splendidly motivated and pay is a crass motivation." In Graham's view, intelligence and altruism are traits that can be passed down through donors to improve the human gene pool (Dice 1994). However, as Barbara from TSBC explained in our 1991 interview,

> I think most men do this for the money—we have a recession to thank for that. I think all the time the rationale changes, but that is a key piece in this. Still, you

get a sense from this process that there are major commitments involved as a donor and that they can't take it lightly as "just a job." Because we constantly need updated information from them and ongoing blood tests, so it's pretty involved. They deserve to be compensated for that. We pay donors on a sliding scale. The highest rate is forty dollars to fifty dollars for each specimen. It's up to the men how much they want to get paid. Some donors don't want to be paid at all, some want a lot. For some guys they really have a hard time with the concept of selling sperm—that's not why they're doing it—but many of them still need the money.

Two of the sperm banks I studied stated that the purchased sample is "corrupted," tainted, not trustworthy. At TSBC, money is considered to be the main reason why men donate sperm, and this is not necessarily thought to detract from the quality of the product; yet there is still an emphasis on the underlying reason men donate—altruism. This emphasis on donors' desire to help those who cannot have children on their own arises due to its association with the quality of person who donates and, by extension, the quality of his genetic material.

These definitions of altruism are problematic, however—especially since it is genetic material that is being provided. In *The Selfish Gene* (1976), Richard Dawkins argues that there is no true altruism, that all acts that appear altruistic are actually self-serving in terms of maximizing an organism's reproductive potential. Although I find flaws with many of Dawkins's sociobiological arguments—that organisms can be reduced to mere containers attempting to spread their genes—in regard to gamete donation, he may have a point: the entire quest for "altruistically" motivated donors is misguided. Any transaction involving the genetic continuation of an individual through his or her offspring is automatically motivated by a certain degree of reproductive self-interest. Even if financial incentive is removed from such transactions, the genetic incentive can still be powerful enough to render the potential donor untrustworthy should he be the type of person who would lie about his family medical history, alcohol or drug use, sexual practices, and so on. These motivations for financial and genetic payoff are not grounded in altruism. Even donors who do express altruistic motivations, such as wanting to help others have children, still express secondary motivations of wanting to spread their genetic material. In addition, sperm banks that have policies against paying their donors, or that only pay them minimal amounts, could financially benefit by selling consumers a product they got for free. Consequently, the search for "altruistic" donors boils down to a search for men who find the genetic incentive to be more significant than financial incentives.

"ETHNIC SPERM" AND EXPANDING PROFITS

Many sperm banks in the San Francisco Bay Area attempted to appeal to an ethnically diverse market by trying to expand their pool of donors. Donor intelligence, donor altruism, and, in some banks, the willingness to be an identity-release donor all affect the perceived value of sperm for both clients and sperm bank personnel. Having donors from a range of ancestral backgrounds was also considered important, but this demand was difficult to fill. Sperm bank representatives would often talk about the need for "ethnic sperm"—by which they often meant Jewish sperm and sperm from people of color—despite the fact that sperm cells themselves do not contain ethnic identity, and people of Anglo-European descent also have a range of ethnic backgrounds. While use of the term *ethnic* is problematic when it comes to sperm, both people in the industry and people selecting sperm for insemination commonly used it.

The more "ethnic" choices sperm banks have in the donor pool, the higher the chances for increased profits. RGC was not concerned with having a broad range of ethnic options, promoting instead the genetic reproduction of primarily white, upper-middle-class, highly educated scientists. Consequently, its donor pool was a comparatively homogenous group, as were its clients. TSBC and RFHS, however, felt a need to recruit donors who were ethnically diverse, and they often relaxed certain standards—such as the minimum five-foot-nine height requirement—for nonwhite donors. This, again, had to do with the politics, policies, and goals of the individual founders of these banks, as well as higher consumer demand in the Bay Area for sperm from men of color.

Leland specifically made the connection between an ethnically diverse donor pool and profit. He stated,

We have one Chinese donor, everyone else is white. If I could find African American or African donors I would be happy as a clam and I'd be making a lot more money. There's a lot of African American lesbians who are looking for African American donors, but can't find any. . . . Unfortunately there has been a large number of calls over the years from African American heterosexual men who are interested in being donors primarily for money, and I turn them away because we don't pay, and some of them ask pretty rude questions like, "Are there any women there to help you have sex?" . . . We also don't have any Jewish sperm, which is a shame because there are a lot of Jewish lesbians who would love to have Jewish sperm.

It is interesting that there is such a high demand for Jewish sperm donors in Bay Area sperm banks. As Susan Kahn (2000) demonstrates in *Reproducing Jews*, because of strict prohibitions against masturbation for Jewish men, non-Jewish sperm is flown to Israel from the United States for Jewish women to use for insemination. Because Jewish identity is matrilineally located, it is the womb that determines the Jewishness of the child. If a child's ethnic or religious identity is traced through the mother, why would there be such a high demand for Jewish sperm in U.S. sperm banks and among Jewish recipients?

All Bay Area sperm bank representatives discussed their desire to recruit greater numbers of diverse—including Jewish—donors and expressed concern and frustration over the lack of diversity in men who are eligible to become donors. This quest for ethnic sperm is motivated in part by a desire to better meet consumer demand; women desire children who share their own (or their partner's) ethnic identity or phenotypic characteristics. Furthermore, sperm banks with a broader selection of donors will also potentially enjoy higher profits. Ethnicity can be symbolically located (or, as in the case of Israeli Jews, dislocated) within the sperm cell, and is thereby assigned economic and emotional value in reproductive transactions.

What is perceived to reside in the sperm? And how do these notions of semen and sperm affect the ways in which donors are recruited and their products marketed and exchanged? The social value of altruism is translated as being intrinsic to the donor (and hence his sperm), demonstrating how widely shared social values are translated into economic value. The underlying philosophies of two of the sperm banks mentioned here are that altruism, or any number of other socially desirable characteristics, is passed from the sperm to the offspring, and that this trait will favorably affect the social world. These fantasies about what sperm is, and about what sperm passes on, are engaged both by repository personnel and founders and by the women who purchase semen in order to have a child.

The commodification and gifting of semen—a transmitter of genetic material—is a complex process. Donors who receive financial compensation for their sperm are part of a process of exchange in which semen flows in and out of sperm banks in exchange for money. This exchange of money for semen appears to be the primary motivation for becoming a donor. Secondary motivations include wanting to pass down one's genes and wanting to help other people. Of course, a desire to help others cannot be viewed as pure altruism because of the underlying motivation to enhance one's reproductive fitness. The reward for men involved in these transactions, then, is threefold: earning money, passing down one's genes, and satisfying a desire to help others.

REPRODUCTIVE WORKERS AND THE MARKET IN GAMETES

Technological reproduction is a multibillion-dollar-per-year industry (U.S. Congress, Office of Technology Assessment, 1988, 61–71). This industry is not limited to the sale of gametes (semen or ova) but rather includes the entire gamut of conceptive technologies, including a variety of treatments for infertility. Andrew Kimbrell's (1993) book *The Human Body Shop* provides a commentary on the design and commodification of life through the sale of body parts, gametes, and blood. Here, he demonstrates how the market—through technology—is increasingly encroaching on the human body, forcing us to redefine life, death, personhood, and property, usually at the expense of ethics.

Many feminist theorists of the 1970s suggest that married, heterosexual sex is a form of reproductive labor, which subordinates women to men in patriarchal societies (Firestone 1970; Leacock 1972; Rubin 1976, 1984; Sacks 1975). Arlie Hochschild's (1983) discussion of "emotional labor" is a gendered redefinition of what constitutes work, and Hochschild attempts to demonstrate the "exchange value" of women's emotional labor in relation to other forms of labor. Literature on the sex industry has explored how sex work is an income-generating form of labor for women or men that is highly globalized and capitalized (Kempadoo 1998; Allison 1994; Frank 2002).

By focusing primarily on the reproductive work of men, rather than women, I am attempting to provide a different slant on feminist critiques regarding the commodification and objectification of the female body. I propose that reproductive technologies evoke a different form of bodywork—which may or may not include some form of sex or pleasure—in which the procreative aspects of the male body become commodified in ways that parallel sex for profit. Here, the notion of reproductive labor takes on a new meaning and a level of monetary value different from that traditionally applied to female reproductive and sexual labor.

Chuck made the connection between sperm donation and sex work explicit: "There was this urologist there and he ran me through some tests and next thing you know, I was part of his stable. That's what he used to call it. His 'stable.' Kinda sounds like the Mustang Ranch, now that I think about it."

Providing sperm can be seen as a type of work; however, it presents a paradox: sperm donation is work that is reframed as a "gift," and there is an emotional and monetary value connected to a donor's altruistic motivations. People buying sperm want to know that the donor is a "nice guy" and that he is "doing it for the right reasons." They want to be able to tell the future children born from his sperm something good about the man who contributed his genetic material to their life. If a man states on his profile that he is doing it for the money, it is less likely an intended parent will choose him. Also, there are human beings involved. A man who provides sperm may at first not think twice about the process, but down the road, when he learns of children born from his sperm, he may think about them, the parents may think about the donor, and the children born may want some sort of contact.

For a popular donor like Chuck, it was not until he learned how many children had been produced from his sperm donations that he actually thought about the end consequences of his time as a donor:

When they retired me, ten years later, they actually said, "We kind of used you longer than we should have. You were popular and productive." So, over ten years

I had about five hundred donations, and they said—I said, "Just out of curiosity, how many?" "Oh, about fifty." And I know other places say it's like thirty or so.

When they told me that, I started thinking about the kids out there. They wouldn't keep using me if I wasn't successful. And then, when I actually found out how many it was kind of like, it kind of blew my mind. I mean, I could potentially see them on the street in their strollers or something. Or they might seek me out. I had never really thought about that before.

Sperm donors participate in a type of work involving the body in which their ability to bring themselves to climax results in increased financial (or social or genetic) opportunities. Sperm donors can make enough money to pay their rent or other expenses. Another donor, Jake, said being a donor was something he looked forward to every week, and that if he weren't a sperm donor he would probably be much more interested in finding a girlfriend. Although he experienced sperm donation as clinical—rather than sexual or erotic—his sexual needs were still taken care of and he received money in exchange for his semen. He said, "I haven't had a girlfriend for quite a while. I mean, if I was dating somebody I probably wouldn't go at all or very rarely, I can imagine. So, yeah, I don't think it's affected my dating life but at the same time I haven't really had time to pursue one much. I don't know. I'm kind of picky about who I want to spend time with. If I did find a girl, I don't think I would probably go there as often." For Jake, sperm donation provided a sexual relief that he would otherwise seek out in a relationship. Sperm donation could possibly be getting in the way of having a fulfilling romantic life.

Reproductive work and sex work are both forms of labor involving the body, where the body or what it produces has a market value. I am using this notion of "reproductive work" as a conceptual category in order to think about the commodification of bodily practices and substances, as well as possible parallels with the sex industry. Semen donors, to my knowledge, do not refer to themselves as "reproductive workers" in the same way that people who provide sex for pay often call themselves "sex workers." Like workers in the sex industry, reproductive workers submit their bodies to a variety of intrusions. Men are subjected to various tests of their semen, urine, urethral cultures, and blood, for which they must be able to perform the sexual act of masturbation, and they must agree to a variety of physical examinations. For women who sell ova, this invasion of bodily boundaries is even more profound. They, too, must agree to physical examinations, including pelvic exams, medical tests for sexually transmitted diseases, and so on, and, if accepted, they are further subjected to hormonal regulation and follicle stimulation and extraction, but without any sexual pleasure. The sexuality of egg donors is more present in how they are visually presented and advertised to appeal to consumers, but not in the egg donation process itself.

CONCLUSION

The business of sperm "donation" presents a paradox: while, on the one hand, it can be perceived as a type of job that one gets paid for, on the other hand, men have complicated reasons for becoming donors that are not always necessarily related to money. Sperm providers can have a mix of these motivations. The focus on altruism is an attempt to remove such "donations" from the realm of market transactions in order to imbue them with a higher meaning. This is an example of what Marx (1906) calls the transcendent quality of a commodity.

The sperm-banking industry's framing that emphasizes altruism is an attempt to decommodify the commodity—to remove semen's status as a marketable product and redefine it as gift, in a way that resonates with deeper cultural moralities. However, representations of reproductive workers in businesses involved in selling their services—which accentuate donor sexuality and the exchange of money for a product—make the argument that gametes are altruistically given gifts untenable, unless gametes are provided without compensation.

Culturally and emotionally, we do not want to think about children as products. The language emphasizing donor altruism is an attempt to imbue sperm donation with a higher moral and emotional value, and to remove these donations from the self-serving commodity culture prevalent in the United States. This is problematic on a deep cultural level, for what is seen as being more self-serving than masturbation—especially for money? Hence, a problem arises in conceptualizing sperm donation: Is it an altruistically given gift that stands above commodity culture, or is it a commodity that is bought, sold, and fetishized? In sperm donation, I argue, "altruism" or "gifting" becomes a selling point, a secondary commodity.

Studying the linkages between cultural values, lay interpretations of genetics, and the market for genetic material is essential to an understanding of how sperm repositories recruit and screen potential donors, why donors provide sperm, and how women choose donors for their offspring and construct the identities of the donors they have chosen. Screening procedures within the sperm-banking industry reflect widely held cultural assumptions surrounding who is and is not suited to reproduce, or, to get more microscopic, which "genes"—and I use the term loosely here—are and are not suited for replication.

Although many in the sperm bank industry contend that men who receive money for sperm are more likely to lie about their health and sexual practices, they fail to recognize that men may have many complicated reasons for donating sperm—that the rewards of genetic continuation and the formation of relationships with children without having to assume responsibility can be even more important than financial compensation. Thus the perceived value and trust in "altruistically donated" sperm is misplaced. In selling sperm (and selling eggs), true altruism—where an individual has no financial or genetic interest—cannot exist.

7 · FROM "OLD EGGS" TO "ODYSSEUS'S JOURNEY"

The Phenomenology of Infertility

Monica always wanted to carry a child and I didn't. I wanted to be a parent but I never had a desire to carry a child. That just didn't fit with who I am. She had four miscarriages. It was awful. After the last one, we were both crying. She couldn't do it anymore and she talked me into trying to do IVF [in vitro fertilization] with her egg. So we tried that twice and I couldn't get pregnant. Then it hit me: being infertile and being lesbian is like a double whammy! I mean, maybe there's something with my body, or something, that makes me butch and infertile.

—Lisa, thirty-eight, with Monica, thirty-six

I really feel like a loss of control over my body, like it's not doing what it is supposed to. I went to law school. I passed the bar. I was in school in psychology. I passed the licensing exams. I take challenges. Like hurdles you run up to them, you jump over them. You take something on and you succeed. And so I thought getting pregnant would be like everything else I've accomplished. But it isn't. I have a horrible image of what it is to be a woman at forty-two trying to get pregnant, not getting pregnant, not having children.

—Rebecca, forty-two

Involuntary childlessness, or infertility, can radically change the way a woman perceives and experiences her body. As Gay Becker demonstrates, infertility has a profound effect on a person's gender identity: For men, infertility is akin to "cutting off your balls" (1990, 1). Women feel as though they have been betrayed by their bodies and masculinized.[1] For gender-nonconforming people, there can be a spectrum of gendered responses. Gender definitions and feelings of femininity are problematic. Some lesbian women who are trying to conceive report feeling like less of a woman in the same way that heterosexual women do. Others report feeling more masculine to begin with, whether it is their partners who are trying to conceive or themselves. Wherever one situates oneself on the gender identity spectrum, infertility still undermines one's sense of self and confidence in one's body to do "what it is supposed to do." Those who identify more as "butch" and are trying to conceive may feel even more marginalized by infertility.

I do not intend to essentialize the biological or "natural" binary categories of male and female. Not all lesbians identify as either feminine or butch, and not all people with female genitalia identify as women. Not all people who identify as women have a deep, burning desire to experience pregnancy. But for those who are trying to conceive—both men and women—infertility represents failure, which is usually interpreted in gendered terms. In the face of this kind of bodily failure, people blame themselves and look for possible causes of their suffering, whether it is promiscuity in their youth, drug use, sexual orientation, or some other possible explanation. Some women I interviewed endured years of unsuccessful attempts to conceive a child but still persisted—spending thousands of dollars and suffering months of anguish—with the hope of someday succeeding.

For most of the women I interviewed, adoption was rarely considered an option and was viewed as a last resort. It is not only the biological relationship to the child that is important but also a compelling desire not to miss out on the experiences of pregnancy and birth, to experience what a woman's body is "supposed to" be able to experience. Throughout this chapter I will illuminate how women experience their bodies and the world around them when numerous attempts to conceive fail to produce a child.

Some women will go to great lengths to have a biological child. Many find themselves seduced by the possibility that another technology, or another drug, or another doctor, or a variety of alternative therapies will help them get pregnant. Most women go beyond the limits they initially set for themselves when they first decided to have a child. This is true for most women trying to conceive, regardless of sexual orientation or marital status. The quest for a biological child can be a long and torturous journey that often fails to lead to the desired result.

MEDICAL VERSUS SOCIAL INFERTILITY AND ACCESS TO CARE

The resources I give out to single straight women and heterosexual couples come out of the gay and lesbian community. It's like, "Thank you very much." We're the ones who normalized donor insemination, because we do things differently than other sperm banks do by providing access to everyone. But I see women all the time who can't get fertility treatment. And it comes down to geographics—even Modesto is different than the Bay

Area. And what we're doing is political. But it's not that radical. I don't get
that whole "family values" thing.

—Geo, health worker at the Sperm Bank of California

Women without male partners seeking infertility treatment faced numerous
obstacles to getting care. In the 1990s and early 2000s, most insurance plans did
not cover infertility treatment, but even those that did certainly did not cover
unmarried women. Since same-sex marriage was not legally recognized, this meant
lesbian couples were denied as well. Insurers—and most physicians throughout
the United States—made a distinction between "medical infertility" and "social
infertility."

Medical infertility was defined as unsuccessful attempts to conceive for a year
or more through heterosexual sex. Medical infertility was considered to be due
to problems with the female reproductive system, the male reproductive system,
a combination of both, or unknown etiology. Social infertility, on the other hand,
was a result of not having "natural access to sperm." Some treatments for medical
infertility were covered, such as surgery to remove fibroids or clear blocked tubes.
Social infertility was not covered at all, unless a physician discovered a woman
had an underlying medical problem. In 1999, only the state of Massachusetts had
a mandate requiring insurers to cover infertility treatment, and this mandate made
a distinction between "medical" and "social" infertility. Medical infertility was covered; social fertility was not. For most women without male partners, traditional
definitions of infertility posed a problem. In order to get an infertility diagnosis,
they had to have been trying unsuccessfully to conceive for a year or more. When
someone is buying sperm, the costs add up quickly. One vial of semen was selling
for around $150 in the 1990s, and most people would buy at least two vials so they
could do two inseminations when they ovulated. Now that same vile of semen
can cost over $800.

Before she started inseminating, Heather had some tests done to make sure she
was reproductively healthy. "I was pretty promiscuous when I was young and with
little or no birth control, so I figured things wouldn't happen quickly, and I wanted
to make sure I would be able to conceive before we spent all that money," Heather
told me. Everything on her exam appeared normal, so they started the insemination process. A year later, Heather had still not gotten pregnant. For Stephanie
(thirty-two) and Heather (twenty-nine), like many lesbian couples, the drawn-out
process of trying to conceive with donor sperm—before becoming eligible for an
infertility diagnosis—was far more costly than it is for straight couples. I spoke
with Heather and Stephanie at their Oakland cottage in May of 1998:

HEATHER: So the infertility work-up, the medical tests, and doctors' appointments,
those were all covered by my insurance. But the sperm and the inseminations, those

were all out-of-pocket. And we tried for a year with donor sperm, and we were spending almost $500 a month on sperm and that adds up! That's $6,000 in a year in sperm and we're still not pregnant! We really needed the insurance to kick in.

STEPHANIE: And the emotional stress. I had a friend who is in a straight relationship. She and her husband had been trying and she had endometriosis, so she has been through some of the same screening and treatments as Heather. The difference is the cost. Ours cost immediately. So when a doctors says, "Why don't you just relax and have a vacation," that doesn't work for us. How do you relax when your legs are up on a table and you have a doctor with a needle going into your cervix, and you're going to have to write a $500 check on your way out?

HEATHER: So yeah, finally after a year of trying with donor sperm and having it fail month after month, and we didn't know if we could keep going because of the emotional and financial toll. So finally after a year of that I had an "infertility diagnosis" and they did a laparoscopy and found out I had endometriosis, and they did some surgeries to fix that problem, which was covered. Then they started putting me on fertility drugs, like HCG and Clomid and they wanted to do IUIs [intrauterine inseminations].[2]

STEPHANIE: But her insurance, I think it was HealthNet, wouldn't cover IUIs with donor sperm—only with a husband's sperm. So we kept trying to fight that and kept getting denied. For lesbian couples you have to pay so much more and wait for more time to pass before you can even get a diagnosis. I read the average amount of time it takes for a lesbian couple to conceive is eighteen months—that's eighteen months of buying frozen sperm, and it's not even the same quality as fresh sperm.

HEATHER: Everything about this process makes you feel so out of control. You're at the mercy of your body, the mercy of the doctors and whether or not they'll treat you, and then at the mercy of the insurance companies. Sometimes we think about adopting, but who is going to let a lesbian couple adopt a kid?

Medical definitions of infertility were based on heteronormative assumptions surrounding reproduction and did not fit the reproductive realities facing women without male partners. In heterosexual couples, the sperm is free. For people using sperm bank donors, the costs start adding up right away. Yet every single woman I spoke to who had difficulty conceiving—regardless of relationship status or sexual orientation—was told by her doctor that she had to be trying for a year or more before she could be diagnosed with infertility, forcing her to waste both precious time and money.

Elaine (fifty-one) and Lynn (thirty-eight) were both Jewish and were looking for a Jewish sperm donor. Although Lynn was the one trying to conceive, Elaine often caught herself thinking about their potential child possibly having blue eyes, like others in her family, forgetting for a moment that she was not contributing her own genetic material to her partner's potential pregnancy. For many same-sex couples attempting to conceive, there is either a forgetting or a sense of grief about not being able to have a biological child together. Over the course of a year, Elaine and Lynn spent $7,000 in sperm and were inseminating with IUIs, performed in the doctor's office.

After a number of early miscarriages, Lynn went to a fertility clinic and told them about the miscarriages, as well as some spotting she had been having for several years, even before she started trying to conceive. The physician at the fertility clinic requested an ultrasound and discovered she had uterine polyps, which were most likely causing her miscarriages.

ELAINE: The interesting thing is, when we went back to our doctor, she said, "Oh, don't worry. You haven't even been trying for a whole year. I wouldn't even consider you infertile until you've been trying for a year." I wanted to say, "Wait a minute. The typical heterosexual couple isn't what we're doing here." For a long time, she was just telling us everything is fine. And I feel bad that I collaborated in that, not wanting to pathologize things. Now we finally know she has polyps that were essentially aborting the pregnancies early.

LYNN: And if we had known that earlier, and had the polyps removed before we started trying, who knows? We could have had a baby by now. Now we're out all this money, wasted all this time, and went through this emotional roller coaster.

ELAINE: For women using sperm donors there really needs to be a more extensive work-up to begin with because we don't have the same situation that heterosexual couples have. But these doctors all operate under a different set of assumptions.

Medical guidelines defining infertility according to the standards for heterosexual couples clearly delayed many women in getting the infertility diagnosis and treatment they needed. Elaine and Lynn were eventually able to get a diagnosis, though, and continue seeking treatment at a fertility clinic after Lynn's surgery to remove the polyps. They went on to do several more IUI cycles after the polyps were removed, but unfortunately they were never able to conceive.

For many unmarried women and lesbian couples, getting access to fertility treatment was extremely difficult, as many medical providers refused to treat them. This led some women to find ways around the obstacles to get the medical care they needed. Gloria (thirty-four) and Dawn (thirty-seven) lived in Atlanta, Georgia. I spoke with them both over the phone, in 1992. They first met at a support group for lesbians who were trying to conceive when they were each with a different partner. Dawn had been trying to conceive for over eight months with her former partner. Gloria had been trying to have a baby with her former partner for over a year without success, suffering repeated miscarriages. Due to Gloria's miscarriages, they decided Dawn should be the one to try to get pregnant first, even though she was older. They had exhausted all their options with Dawn's regular ob-gyn and now wanted to seek treatment with a fertility specialist.

DAWN: So we did a GIFT[3] procedure at the University of Alabama, because they didn't care if we were married or not, but we had to travel a long distance, and that was really trying. When that failed we decided we couldn't keep going that distance every month. But here in Atlanta, the doctor that I had been seeing, his partners wouldn't approve my being a participant in the IVF program unless I had a husband. . . . So I said, "OK, I have one."

DIANE: How did you do that?

DAWN: I bought one. It was kind of creepy, you know, to have to lie like that. But when we were referred to this doctor, the woman who referred us was a counselor at a feminist women's health center here, where we could be open. But she advised us not to be open to this particular group of doctors. So any time Gloria went with me she was just my "friend."

We had this gay friend and we knew beforehand that he didn't have a sperm count that was compatible with fertility. So he agreed to be a stand-in husband but didn't have to be a stand-in donor. We could get another donor. His presence wasn't required once his sperm tests came back unusable.

GLORIA: They encouraged Dawn to have her significant other or husband present, so we took that as an invitation for me to be there, without really telling them anything about our relationship. They probably knew, but it wasn't any of their business anyway. They said she had to have a husband, so she had one. Going through that process, we decided we wanted to get married, so we had a ceremony on Pride Day. It's not legally recognized in Georgia, but we wanted that commitment to each other.

Getting affordable access to treatment posed numerous challenges for women without male partners. For women like Stephanie and Heather—who need donor sperm to conceive—costs added up substantially before they were able to get an infertility diagnosis. This was also true for Elaine and Lynn, whose physician followed the standard definitions of infertility, refused to do a fertility work-up, and delayed Lynn in getting the diagnosis that might have improved her chances of conceiving—if she had not waited too long. This is a burden women with male partners do not face.

Insurance coverage for infertility treatment is notoriously problematic for everyone, regardless of sexual orientation or marital status. However, all women attempting to conceive on their own or with a female partner faced hurdles in getting insurance to pay for portions of their infertility treatment that are routinely covered for heterosexual couples. Some women, like Dawn and Gloria, were forced to circumvent discriminatory clinic policies by lying to their doctors and finding creative ways to get access to medical care. The Ethics Committee of the American Society for Reproductive Medicine (ASRM) now recommends that lesbians, gay men, and unmarried persons have the right to be parents and be granted access to fertility treatment, but this recommendation was not made until

2013 (Ethics Committee of the ASRM 2013). In 2015, the committee (Ethics Committee of the ASRM 2015) issued a similar opinion on the right of transgender people to have access to fertility treatment.

INFERTILITY AS ODYSSEUS'S JOURNEY

When women—lesbian, straight, or bisexual, single or with a partner—experience infertility, they often describe their path to parenthood as a type of heroine's journey, filled with challenges and struggles. The metaphors they use to describe their bodies, their relationship to the medical establishment, and how infertility affects their relationships with their lovers illustrate the emotional conflicts infertility raises in their lives. Going through this process can be extremely taxing on relationships, especially if both members of the couple have different priorities surrounding having a child. And many women, regardless of their sexual orientation, stay in relationships too long, hoping they can convince their partner to come around to the idea of trying for a baby. For many, the time spent waiting is time spent wasting their fertile years—until they vanish.

Before she met her current partner, Janine (thirty-seven), Becky (forty-one) spent five years in a relationship with another woman, hoping she could change her mind about trying to have a child:

> I started raising this issue with her that I wanted to have a child and she was vehemently opposed to it. We struggled around this one issue for many years—until I was about thirty-five or thirty-six—and I was about to have a gay male friend of mine be the donor and co-parent. Suddenly, she broke up with me, and I was devastated but I decided to have a child on my own.
>
> Then I met another woman who asked me to wait six months to see if we really wanted to be together. I had been about to start and then she said she didn't like the donor I had chosen, so she and I looked for another donor. And then I did get pregnant in about six months, but it was what they call a "blighted ovum" and I had to have a DNC [abortion]. And that led to that breakup because it made it clear for her she didn't want to do this. She did not want to raise a child with me. So I was on my own again.

Like Becky, Rebecca spent years seeking motherhood within relationships. Unlike Becky, she was straight, and searching for the "right man" to have a child with. By the time I met Rebecca in 1997, she had been trying to conceive for three years on her own, but still kept hoping she would find a partner. I asked her how she decided she wanted to have a child on her own, and her story, exhausting, sometimes funny, but overall tragic, virtually poured out during the three and a half hours I was at her home:

When I was thirty-eight, I started thinking about it as something I could never do. I cried all the time. Whenever the subject of babies would come up, I would weep. At that point, I went into a pretty intense quest to find a partner. I did personal ads and dated a zillion people—kind of got compulsive about it.

Then I turned forty, and it really turned up the heat for me. . . . I met a man in Ireland, . . . so I spent about a year hoping and being courted and courting him, and hoping that it would work out, with multiple trips back and forth. . . . At some point I just decided this is it, I have to move forward on this [if I want to get pregnant]. . . .

It was pretty much the end of our relationship. . . . Making the decision to end the relationship was not that difficult. Making the decision to try to inseminate by myself was much harder. . . . It was the idea of doing it alone, not just the reality of doing it without him, but this was going to be me doing it alone, and I had such a strong feeling, especially when I started this process, such an intense feeling of, "This is wrong," or "I'm supposed to do this with a man."

The idea of being a single mother got to be pretty, really amazing, it got to be a real. . . . How can I even describe it? It really felt like quite the spiritual quest when I was wrestling with it. It doesn't feel like that now, but it did very much so then. And, I struggled a lot with, "Could I do it by myself? Would it be OK with my friends and family, if I did it all by myself?" and a lot of sadness about not having it be the ideal way, not having it be the storybook way. It's amazing, but there was a period when it was like walking on a very thin path, and on either side of you is this enormous ravine, and if you take a step off either side, you fall into the ravine, and there are flames, and it's like you're drowning, you know, it's overwhelming, you know?

Rebecca's story depicts some common themes among single women trying to conceive a child on their own: the desire to have a child *with* someone becomes a driving force in their relationships—often leading to a series of failed relationships; women often hold on to the relationship, thinking they will be able to convince their partner to pursue parenthood with them—even when the partner explicitly states that he or she is not interested in having a child; and the idea of having a child on one's own can seem so overwhelming that many invest precious time in relationships until the clock runs out.

Cultural stories about meeting "the One" and having the ideal family pervade many women's thinking on the subject of having children, and this results in a great deal of conflict and sadness when these stories fail to be actualized in women's own lives. In both straight and lesbian relationships, the idea of having a child on one's own can be so overwhelming for women that they delay or interrupt their attempts to conceive a child when faced with a new relationship—especially if the partner is uncertain about having children. Sometimes the new relationship buckles under the pressure of the woman's quest to have a child.

And the journey is a long road for many women once they begin the donor insemination process. Rebecca continued,

> So, I made the decision and I started it. The sperm bank was called. The thing was set up. I started. At the beginning I was convinced I was going to be pregnant. And the first three times I did it, I was sure I was pregnant each time. I was really pretty naive about it.
>
> And the people at the sperm bank told me I ought to do the inseminations through them. I should do two a month and I should do one at home and one with them. So that's how I did it. And I paid. I was feeling flush with money at that point. I was paying cash at that point because I didn't even have an infertility diagnosis until six months into the process. I was paying cash for the insemination.

When repeated attempts at self-insemination did not result in pregnancy, most women, including Rebecca, opted to seek treatment through an infertility specialist. What first appears to be a new solution to the problem of getting pregnant often becomes a new set of challenges and struggles. Rebecca described her experience:

> By about my fifth or sixth cycle, I was doing the inseminations through my doctor. Then she went on pregnancy leave without even telling me. I couldn't believe it, I went in there for the insemination and she was clearly pregnant and the next time I went in, she was gone. Then cycle seven or eight another doctor in that office, said, "If you want to get pregnant, you shouldn't be here. We just can't provide you with the kind of infertility treatment you need."
>
> So, I went to Dr. Borovski's office and I did a stimulated cycle with him using Fertinax, which is, you know, the easy injection form of Pergonal and did not respond well to it. My estrogen level had gone up. I got one nice-sized follicle and one small, maybe inconsequential follicle, and Dr. Borovski said, "You flunked." That's what he said. "Well, I have to say you flunked this test." He was awful.
>
> So, I did a second cycle with him, and then I did a third one with him. And, you know, I was talking with him about what other kind of drugs that I might try, or what else he would recommend, and he basically said, "Well, I don't think you'll do very well on any of them." And basically said to me after the insemination, "You know, you have to stop doing this." And, I said, "What do you mean?" Nobody had given me a diagnosis. But he said, "Well, you have reduced ovarian capacity, and your age, and you're not producing any eggs, you only got one good egg, and you flunked the test." He said it again. Twice he said I flunked. I remember that. Because, it was like water in the face.
>
> You know, the whole process is so emotional. It's really hard to remember that you're just talking with technicians, like auto mechanics, and they have no existential advice to give you about the process. They just tell you whether they think

that, you know, you can straighten out this chassis after a big car crash. And, he said to me, you know, "You should do donor egg," and I said, "Well, that's a big step, that's a big different deal." And, he said, "Yeah, it's just like adopting, but you'll get pregnant and you get to puff out, and waddle around, and you know, you feel like you're pregnant." That's exactly how he said it.

Early on, it really felt like, you know, Odysseus's journey. You're on a boat, and there are things on either side, and there are one-eyed monsters, and that doctor, Dr. Borovski, was definitely my Cyclops. So, the next insemination he wouldn't do.

You know, one thing about this process is it has completely changed how I view doctors. I think they're really awful. I think they're monsters.

Rebecca's story exemplifies many of the issues women face in infertility diagnosis and treatment. The first has to do with the mutual discomfort between doctors who get pregnant and their infertile patients. Rebecca was taken aback, and possibly somewhat resentful, when her doctor was visibly pregnant, and she felt hurt when the doctor failed even to say good-bye. The doctor possibly also felt uncomfortable about addressing her own pregnancy with her infertile patients. Although doctors are not normally compelled to discuss their own conditions with patients, the public nature of pregnancy makes many patients—especially infertile patients—feel as if they are due an explanation. Second, this doctor's replacement suggested that Rebecca seek help elsewhere if she wanted to conceive, despite the fact that this office specialized in infertility. This doctor let Rebecca know she needed much more invasive treatment than that practice was able to provide if she were going to have any hope of conceiving—news Rebecca did not want to hear.

The conflict between doctor-patient relations is exemplified in Rebecca's encounters with Dr. Borovski. Despite the fact that Dr. Borovski was painfully blunt with her and described her as having "flunked the test" of fertility, Rebecca continued her treatments with him. She was not ready to hear what he was telling her: her chances of conceiving at her age, with her eggs, were minimal. Dr. Borovski's refusal to continue treating Rebecca was, perhaps, an ethical one. Perhaps he did not want her to continue wasting her money on a process he knew would not be successful. However, she wanted to run out of his office and find someone who could tell her what she wanted to hear—that they could help her get pregnant with her own biological child.

Rebecca's analogy of physicians being like auto mechanics is apt. Despite his crassness in broaching the subject of using an egg donor, Dr. Borovski thought in terms of technical solutions to the problem of her infertility. Rebecca, on the other hand, was immersed in the experience of having an infertile body and concerned with the social and biological relationship she would have with a child. This became especially apparent as she discussed her views toward using an egg donor:

You know, if there were a man in my life, I think I would do donor egg now. Maybe take a couple of months off to think about it but without much hesitation, I think I would move in that direction. But the idea of doing donor egg and donor sperm both is off-putting to me. Because, it's like nobody's baby.

One of the reasons I've put myself through this, I'm a little chagrined to admit, there aren't a lot of people who are genetically related to me around. I have a really strong longing to have somebody who has my genetic heritage. I just think it would be really hard for me to have kids without that genetic connection. . . . I would constantly be wondering, like whose nose is that? Is that weird thing that you do, did you get that from somebody, is there somebody else around who does that too?

Rebecca articulated one reason why so many women and couples undergo years of costly infertility treatment: for some, having a child who does not have your (or your partner's) genetic heritage can feel like having "nobody's baby." If the infant is not genetically linked to the parents, then to whom does it belong? When intended parents navigate their way through infertility treatment, and ultimately reach the point where using a donor or a gestational surrogate is their only option (other than adoption) for having a child, the meaning of "own child" shifts in order to accommodate the parents' connection to their child (Melhuus 2012). For example, if a person uses an egg donor and a sperm donor with a gestational surrogate, in order to accept the child as their "own" they need to define the mother as the person who gestates, delivers, and nurtures the child. For someone using their own egg and a gestational surrogate, the parent is the one who has a genetic connection to the child, rather than the gestational connection. For two-mom families, "own child" is not exclusively defined by biology or gestation, but expands to include both the biological (or gestational) mother and the woman who takes on the social role of mothering. Some lesbian couples may have one partner donate eggs to the other so they other can carry and deliver the child; in this way, both mothers have some biological connection—whether genetic or gestational—to strength their connection and legal rights to a child. In order to pursue third-party technological reproduction, a person must first come to terms with the idea that their "own child" is the child they nurture and love, rather than exclusively a child they had a role in creating.

Rebecca is not the only woman I interviewed who perceived the lack of biological connection as a major obstacle to overcome in order to have a child through either donor egg or adoption. Her entire notion of having a child is connected to her idea of the genetic continuity of her family. Her desire to be biologically connected to the child she raises is directly affected by her desire to place herself and whatever offspring she might have within the context of her family, as well as a desire to feel a deeper connection to a father who was not there for her. Having a child, then, is not always just about being a mother per se; it is about re-establishing relationships with and connections to the rest of her family. The experience of infertility, then, goes far beyond the inability to have a child.

For Rebecca, the underlying motivations for trying to have a biological child are connected to her notion that genetic kin have more interconnections within a family—an interesting blend of familiarity and uniqueness. She does not want to have "nobody's baby." She also sees this as important because of her relationship with her own inaccessible father. Finally, she began to think about when she might stop infertility treatment and consider other options, but she expressed deep regret that she did not try to have a child earlier, when her body would have been more likely to conceive.

Rebecca described the struggles she went through: "When I started this process, I thought, 'OK. I'm going to get pregnant.' Now, it's kind of like, 'Oh, my God! Is there any way that I'll get pregnant?' And, what have I made a decision to do? Torture myself? There's like this whole ocean of flaming waves around, you know, hitting me with 'Why didn't I do this earlier?' If I really wanted it, why didn't I do it at a time when I could? If I can want it so much now, why the hell didn't I want to when I could have had it?

The themes Rebecca so vividly described are common among women who navigate through the "flaming waves" of infertility treatment. They focus on aging, relationships, social restrictions, the cost of donor semen and medical treatment, experiences and perceptions of the medical system, notions of the family and genetic relatedness, and coming to terms with failure. These themes are evident throughout other women's stories as well.

PREGNANCY FAILURES AND THE FEMALE BODY

Women who are trying to conceive experience a heightened sense of the body—for example, feeling pregnant after inseminations when it is far too early to detect actual signs of pregnancy like swollen breasts or fatigue. They also experience mood swings from fertility drugs they have to inject into their bodies, lost pregnancies, and heartbreak at the sight of menstrual blood—the marker of another failed attempt to conceive a child. Time is experienced in relation to how many cycles of failed inseminations a woman has endured. And the body—for women who want to conceive and carry a baby to term but cannot—is viewed as the enemy and becomes a source of alienation and failure.

Marla, now forty-six, had wanted a child as long as she could remember. "When I was six, I used to play with my dolls and give them names and think that those would be the names I would give my kids someday," she told me when I visited her at her home in Pacifica. Throughout her adolescence, she had irregular menstrual cycles, but she did not really think much of it until her appearance started changing. By twenty, she started having intermittent spotting and suddenly gained weight, going from about 120 pounds to 140 pounds in a matter of months. She went to the doctor and discovered she had polycystic ovary syndrome (PCOS), and he told her she would likely never be able to conceive and deliver a child.

I was very frightened. Not too long after I saw the doctor, my symptoms started getting worse. I was growing a lot of hair, just turning into a gorilla. I had hair on my face, bushy eyebrows, oily scalp, gaining weight, and at the time I didn't know why. They said I produced too much testosterone, so he put me on birth control pills to regulate my cycle, but the pills didn't do anything for the other symptoms.

When I was in high school, I was attractive. I was social and had a lot of dates. Once the PCOS started hitting me, suddenly guys didn't want to date me anymore. Girls didn't want to hang out with me. I was isolated. I had to start doing electrolysis, fighting the beard growing on the side of my face, using make up, trying to manage the weight gain, and I started dating again in my twenties, but I had to do a lot to look like a woman.

In my twenties, I had a number of relationships, but none of them wanted kids, except for one guy I was with for six months when I was thirty-five. I guess I should have jumped on that deal when I had the chance. But these guys just weren't right. They weren't suitable. I only knew one man who cared about me enough to say, "I know you want to have children," and asked me to have a child with him. But that relationship didn't work out, and with my symptoms getting worse—the hirsutism and weight gain—my options were getting less. I wasn't as attractive as I was before.

It was not too long after we broke up that I found out about sperm banks. A friend sent me an article. I had never heard of donor sperm before. If I had known that was an option, I would have started trying in my twenties, because I knew I would have a difficult time getting pregnant because of all the cysts on my ovaries and my hormones.

So I went to the sperm bank, and I didn't care about hair color or height or any of those things. I just wanted someone with good, healthy sperm. And I'm very grateful to these donors who have so willingly given a part of their body to me. I mean, they've given me a part of their life, their genes, you know? And I know they're getting paid for it, but still, it's a huge sacrifice. I had never had such a gift before.

So I was really happy to have that. The doctor put me on Clomid. And I thought they had figured out how to regulate my system, my hormones, properly. And I got pregnant at forty-one, but four and a half months later I had a miscarriage. I was rushed to the hospital with this umbilical cord coming out of me and they told me she was dead. My whole life fell apart. I haven't been able to get pregnant again since.

But even being devastated by losing her, I'm happy I got to know her at four and a half months. That was the most precious time of my life. I still have the ultrasound pictures of the footprints and everything. I'm thankful for that. And for that short amount of time, my body, I felt like a normal woman.

So now, on top of the polycystic ovaries, I've got old eggs. Having a child? That door is closed to me. And I've got these cysts all over my ovaries, and my doctor says he needs to take them out, and that will throw me right into menopause. The polycystic ovaries have been a living hell for me. I have ongoing pain in my ovary. I look like a man. I have weight gain, horrible acne, a sleep disorder. They're all part of it. PCOS has devastated my life. I think removing my ovaries at this point will probably be a relief. They've done nothing but cause me grief.

Marla's experience as a woman with PCOS has completely derailed her sense of self, her self-esteem, and her feelings about her body. Not only did she feel marginalized because of how PCOS affected her looks, and masculinized in a body that had previously felt feminine, but she also felt alienated by the body that failed her in her attempts to realize her lifelong dream to be a mother. Her only experience of motherhood, and the only time since adolescence that she truly felt like "a normal woman," was in those brief four and a half months when she was pregnant, before she lost her much-wanted daughter. She feels betrayed by her body, which turned her life into "a living hell."

Some women blame themselves for their inability to conceive and see it as being connected to emotional issues related to trauma. Heather, for example, explained her infertility in light of having been molested as a child: "I was molested by my stepfather for six years from the age of twelve until I left home at eighteen. And going through all this trauma with infertility treatment, I started thinking, maybe I can't get pregnant because of emotional blocks from having been molested, like I closed off my body and I wasn't receptive. So I started seeing an acupuncturist and a shaman. So the shaman and I were looking at the issues of the incest and being molested for as many years as I was and just how that might sabotage emotionally the feeling around wanting a child."

For Heather, infertility was emotionally linked to having been victimized by someone she should have been able to trust, leaving her to feel closed off and blocking emotional intimacy as well as bodily receptivity. While there could have been trauma to her body that interfered with her ability to conceive, she perceives the trauma as the cause of an emotional block and takes the blame for sabotaging herself. Furthermore, she told me that she was a DES (diethylstilbestrol) daughter—a far more likely cause of her infertility.[4] Heather's tendency toward self-blame and belief that she suffers from an emotional block that prevents her from opening up to pregnancy are responses also seen in other women going through infertility—especially women who have experienced sexual trauma.

Women suffering from infertility often view their bodies in negative terms. They discuss their bodies in terms of failure, and most often perceive this failure as directly connected to their femininity or wholeness as women. In fact, women who are attempting to conceive typically discuss their concern that they have "old eggs" or that the "eggs have gone bad." These images of the internal body as old, dried up, useless, and empty pervaded throughout my conversations with women experiencing infertility, as well as with some who simply took longer than expected to conceive. Most women trying to conceive typically share the idea that conceiving and bearing babies is something the female body is supposed to do, and if the body fails in this task, one is "less of a woman" and probably only has oneself to blame. For example, Lynn, a thirty-seven-year-old woman living with her female partner, told me her story of infertility:

> I feel like my body has failed me. You start to ruminate about all the things you might have done growing up that might have made it hard for you to have a baby now. Like, I used to party a lot when I was younger. I had an IUD that caused a pelvic infection. . . . Also, I had an abortion when I was twenty-three and that's been a big deal in my mind from a sort of spiritual aspect—am I paying for doing that now? . . . At this point, I don't look back on that as much as I used to, but I think it is definitely hard to keep a good concept of yourself while you're trying to do this. I think I made good decisions when I made them, but I believe in Karma a lot. I don't know how much of that comes into play here.

Self-blame is common among women experiencing infertility. Several women told me they thought their infertility could be attributed to "having partied too much" when younger; one informant who was single stated she felt her infertility was because she should not be trying to have a baby on her own.

These tendencies toward self-blame are typically connected with the notion of Karma—that something one has done in the past, or has been done to one in the past, or whom one decided to have sexual relations with, or the number of sexual partners one has had, explains one's inability to conceive a child. Typically, women described their physical bodies (i.e., their reproductive organs) as being somehow blocked, emotionally or psychically, by the events that have occurred in their lives. These magical explanations are especially pronounced when no explanation has been given to women regarding the medical reasons for their infertility. The types of therapies many women seek for infertility treatment are consistent with many women's interpretations of infertility within a sort of cosmic etiology.

The medical journey through infertility treatment is an arduous one, emotionally, financially, and physically. It is marked not only by bodily failures but also by increasing medical management and bodily invasions as one treatment after another leaves one empty-handed. After regular donor insemination fails repeatedly, the next step would be to try IUI. Different fertility drugs, such as Clomid, Pergonal, Menopur, and Follistim, may be used to stimulate the ovaries to produce more eggs than usual or to improve egg quality in order to increase the likelihood of conception, or progesterone may be used to help prevent miscarriage. Some of these drugs can have dramatic effects on emotions and can have physical side effects as well. But starting down the infertility treatment path, people always hold out the hope that a different drug, or the next level of medical treatment, will produce the desired result. Many people, whether in same-sex relationships, on their own, or in heterosexual relationships, have a difficult time deciding when to stop, and they may end up pursuing options they never thought they would when they first started on this journey. These things are stressful and can affect people's relationships.

Gretta (thirty) and Ruth (thirty-three) first met in Europe in 1992, when they were both in their late twenties. They moved to California the following year, and Gretta, as she tells it, starting getting "obsessed" about starting a family. "The whole biological clock thing really hit me," she said. "I mean we'd see babies in restaurants and I would be like 'Oh my God I want one.' Ruth had to stop me from going over and picking them up out of their high chairs." When they started trying to conceive, Gretta went to the doctor for an exam and discovered she was not ovulating, so the doctor put her on Clomid and they started home inseminations.

GRETTA: So we started with home inseminations, [but] it just wasn't working. So after about six months of that we talked the doctor into starting IUI. She wanted to wait until we had been trying a year without success, but we talked her into the IUI right away. When you're buying sperm, you just don't have that kind of time and money.

RUTH: And the Clomid, that was really hard. She was like a completely different person. I mean, it's kind of funny sometimes, but . . .

GRETTA: Yeah, we kind of joke about my "Clomid moments."

RUTH: The joke last time was, Gretta was putting away a dish of lasagna in the fridge and she set it down on something hot, with cellophane on top. And I said something like, "That doesn't look like a very good place for it." And she mocked me and said, "That doesn't look like a good place for it," in kind of a nasty tone.

GRETTA: Suddenly I just snapped, and I stormed past her and I picked up the lasagna pan and I hurled it at the wall. I'm not usually the kind of person to throw things, but I just threw the entire dish. There was lasagna all over the wall and I was just standing in the midst of it, with broken Pyrex on the floor, weeping. I think there was even lasagna in my hair. Ruth got quickly out of the kitchen and came back a few minutes later and goes: "Are you having a Clomid moment?" [Both laugh.]

Gretta and Ruth continued to describe their anxiety about home insemination:

RUTH: She wanted me to inseminate her and I really had a lot of anxiety about that. Kind of like performance anxiety. My stomach would get tied up in knots and I'd almost get sick. I mean on the one hand, there I am having to deal with this sperm, and as a lesbian all my life, I never had to deal with sperm. It was just weird. And

then at the same time there's all this pressure, like I'm supposed to get her pregnant and if I don't I'm failing as her partner.

DIANE: So it wasn't romantic at all?

GRETTA: God no. I was doing these ovulation kits trying to time my ovulation. And
then we read somewhere that it's better if you have an orgasm if you're trying to
conceive, and we were like, "What? How am I supposed to have an orgasm when
we're sitting there with a vial of sperm, I just checked my kit to make sure it's the
right time, she's about to vomit because of her performance anxiety and dealing
with this sperm, and I've got my legs in the air asking, "Did you put in yet?"

RUTH: So not sexy! I think we were both relieved when we finally moved to IUI.
Then it was out of our hands. It was more clinical, and more inconvenient, but a
lot less anxiety.

GRETTA: Yeah, now I'm on Clomid and HCG [human chorionic gonadotropin] and
doing another IUI next week. If that doesn't work, we'll start having to think about
the next steps.

Women being treated for infertility not only experiment with the broad range
of available biomedical therapies but also seek help from a variety of complemen-
tary indigenous and alternative therapists. For example, several women told me
of the Chinese herbs they drink that "taste like piss." During my interview with
Rebecca, she discussed her visits to numerous medical practitioners, a therapist
to help her with her mental block against conceiving, her acupuncturist, and her
Chinese herbalist. When asked why she saw so many different practitioners for
this one problem, she explained that it made her feel as though she was taking
action—that it gave her some control in a situation in which she felt she had none.
The need to have some control over one's treatment, when one feels one has no
control over the ability of one's body to conceive a child, was typical among the
women I interviewed.

Physicians, too, prescribe therapies that are more like traditional and indigenous medicine than what we have come to know as allopathic medicine. For example, Rebecca told me, "I remember one thing that was hysterically funny. One
doctor wanted to give me cocoa butter suppositories, instead of progesterone,
because the progesterone was giving me yeast infections. So I thought, 'Great!
Cocoa butter suppositories.' But it drips out of you; it makes you smell like a
banana split. It's the weirdest thing. It makes you smell like a hot fudge sundae.
And there have been just so many moments like that, you wonder what next? I'm
a banana split in service of this fertility thing."

Thus, the woman undergoing infertility treatment is "in service" to her desire
to have a child and will put her body through varied treatments in order to achieve
this goal. The body, for these women, is viewed as something that has failed them
and has diminished their feelings of self-worth. Women undergoing infertility,

then, feel alienated from their own bodies. However, these same bodies are also typically viewed as somehow being victims of mental or emotional blocks impeding their ability to open up to allow conception to occur.

THE PHENOMENOLOGY OF FAILED PREGNANCY

Many women are able to conceive but experience repeated pregnancy loss and are seemingly unable to carry a child to term. For those who have suffered repeated miscarriages, the body is not usually viewed as "blocked," as it is among women who have not been able to conceive. However, the sense of failure and loss of control of the body is more profound.

Janine and Becky lived in separate residences but spend their time in each household with Andrea, Janine's three-year-old daughter through donor insemination. Becky was attempting to have a child through donor insemination but has had numerous miscarriages. She first started trying to have a child in a former relationship, which broke up following her first miscarriage. After that relationship failed, she decided to have a child on her own. She then met Janine, when Janine was seven months pregnant. Becky had been a steady presence in Andrea's life and planned on adopting her through second-parent adoption. Becky discussed how she decided to use a known donor and described her experiences with pregnancy and miscarriage:

> I started inseminating almost three years ago, when I was involved with another lover. It took me six months to get pregnant, and the relationship was getting really rocky. But I got pregnant, and as far as I knew, everything was OK. Then I decided to get a CVS [chorionic villi sampling], instead of an amniocentesis, when I was about nine weeks pregnant, and they told me there was nothing there. So they had to perform a DNC [abortion]. I had what they call a "blighted ovum." I was completely devastated, but I figured a lot of women have one miscarriage. But that miscarriage precipitated the final breakup of my relationship with my lover. She decided she just did not want to do this, did not want to raise another child.
>
> Anyway, so I got pregnant again two months after my miscarriage. This time, again, everything seemed to be going OK, but suddenly I didn't feel pregnant anymore. I could just tell by the way my breasts felt. My doctor wanted me to come in around ten weeks to see if they could hear the heartbeat. So I went in and they couldn't hear it. Everyone tried to say, "Oh, just relax and everything will be fine," but they sent me for a sonogram. I went for the sonogram, and this time it wasn't a blighted ovum, but it was dead. I couldn't believe it!
>
> That was just before my fortieth birthday. I waited three months to try again, and this time I didn't get pregnant right away. It's really hard when you're inseminating. You can't just wait and see what happens. You have to be really purposeful about it: you take your temperature, chart everything, think about what kind of

cervical mucus you're producing, and try to decide whether you should do it today, or tomorrow, in the morning or in the afternoon.

When I was trying to get pregnant the third time, that's when Janine and I became involved. It took me six months to get pregnant this time, and I was very anxious when I got pregnant the third time, and the doctor agreed to do a sonogram at seven weeks to see if we could see the heartbeat, and said we'd use progesterone suppositories to help prevent miscarriage. So at seven and a half weeks I went and they saw a heartbeat. They said everything looks fine. I was completely amazed, but I relaxed a little bit. I started feeling pregnant again. So, I got to eleven weeks and I thought, "Maybe I'm actually going to do it this time. Maybe I'm actually going to make it to the second trimester." I felt like if I could make it that far I could relax. Then at eleven and a half weeks, on a Sunday, I just suddenly started bleeding, and the doctor said I should stay on bed rest and go in for a sonogram on Monday. And they did a sonogram, and once again it was dead.

There was no explanation. This miscarriage was completely devastating to me. There was like this cumulative emotional effect—it was just awful. Then I decided to change donors because I thought maybe my donor and I were genetically a bad match, or something. It was really hard for me to change donors because I'd become really attached to him, and to the idea of using a known donor. But I also felt I had to make sure I tried everything to avoid having another miscarriage. So Janine set up everything with the sperm bank for me. So I started inseminating again, and had my fourth miscarriage when I was about six weeks pregnant. This time I wasn't quite as upset as the time before, though. I mean, I never had the chance to see the heartbeat during this last pregnancy—I never had the chance to really believe in it.

But, pregnancy has totally changed its meaning for me. Now when I inseminate, it's like, you have those two weeks to wait to find out if you're pregnant. On top of that, if I am pregnant there's the three weeks to wait before you find out if you've got a heartbeat. I see pregnancy in these different stages. But I never get to that milestone where you see the heartbeat and your pregnancy just continues. My perspective is being pregnant means you're very anxious for a few weeks and then you have a DNC. That's my experience of pregnancy. It's strange, I feel very defined by having had four miscarriages. It's always present. In some ways, I don't believe anything else is possible. Having a full-term pregnancy and a baby seems unrealistic or crazy to me. It's sort of this unattainable thing—a fantasy.

For women who experience repeated miscarriages, the body is also perceived as something that fails to do what it is supposed to do. Women express feeling "out of control" and take measures to try to control whatever they can in the process of conceiving or maintaining a pregnancy. Time, again, is perceived in relation to the cycles of the body when one is undergoing insemination. If conception occurs, this perception of time is replaced by one marked by the gestational weeks of the pregnancy, which are viewed as hurdles to jump. Furthermore, there is the perception of feeling pregnant or not feeling pregnant. A woman may actually be pregnant but not feel pregnant because of fears surrounding losing the pregnancy.

Linda Layne's (2003) ethnography, *Motherhood Lost*, provides a deeply personal feminist account of the devastating experience of miscarriage, and demonstrates how pregnancy loss reveals broader social meanings at the margins of life and death. Rayna Rapp's (1999) analysis of fetal imagery provided by ultrasound further illuminates how technologies make a pregnancy seem more real. Technology validates or invalidates pregnancy sensations and heightens the body knowledge of a continuing or lost pregnancy. For women going through infertility treatment—as for other pregnant women—the image of the fetus can provide reassurance that everything is OK, or even joy at having finally succeeded. For women who endure repeated miscarriages, though, this imagery makes the experience of pregnancy loss even more profound. Here, again, a woman feels defined by her experiences of not being able to carry a child to term.

CONCLUSION

Katharine Young's (1997) *Presence in the Flesh* provides an ethnographic account of how the body is inscribed by surgery and how surgery is an experience that forever transforms and defines the body and person. Her analysis certainly resonated with my own experiences with ovarian surgery, but it also made me think about how motherhood and infertility affect body perception and experience. Anthropological discussions of the body also explore issues of gender, culture, and power. Emily Martin (1987) demonstrates how women relate to the dominant cultural categories through their conversations about themselves and their bodily processes. Thomas Laquer (1990), a social historian, explores how social and medical constructs of sex, gender, and the body have changed through time and how seemingly stable categories are actually mutable. The body is seen as a text that can be read: interpretations of the body, gender, and sexuality are situated within a wider sociopolitical context, which is rooted in changing historical circumstances (Flax 1990; Haraway 1991; Bordo 1993). As people navigate through medical settings in search of treatment for infertility, their bodies are scrutinized, defined, inscribed, and sometimes screened out, and their perceptions of self are distorted.

All of the women I spoke to—those who conceived relatively quickly, as well as those who spent years trying unsuccessfully to conceive a child or carry a child to term—discussed how their perceptions of their bodies changed through the process. Women who conceived relatively quickly (within six to nine months) discussed how much more aware they have become of their bodies through the process of charting their temperatures, evaluating the consistency of the cervical mucus to decide when to inseminate, and looking for signs of pregnancy like nausea, breast tenderness, feeling emotional, and so on. For women who spend a year or more trying to have a child—especially those who remain childless—infertility becomes part of their identity, part of how they define themselves and their bodies.

For the most part, women who have endured infertility perceive their bodies as failing to do what they were meant to do. This failure has dramatic consequences for a woman's perception of self. For example, one woman in a lesbian relationship told me how much it defined her as female: "I never was into feminine things, like dresses and makeup and stuff, but this [pregnancy] was something I really wanted—something that I really feel that I am supposed to be able to do." For all women I interviewed who wanted to carry a child, the ability to conceive was directly linked to their identity as a woman. For women in lesbian relationships who did not want to be the one to conceive and deliver a baby, however, this was not considered to be an issue.

For single women, infertility emphasizes the fact that they are alone in the world—a further reminder of failed relationships. Some blamed themselves for staying too long in relationships they knew were doomed to fail but for which they held out hope that things would eventually work out. Marla had underlying hormonal issues that affected both her fertility and her body, causing her to look more masculine, which she felt was a complete gender failure. Though Heather was a DES daughter, which likely caused her inability to have a child, she still blames herself and the fact that she had been molested as a child. For some lesbian couples, infertility has caused the breakup of their relationships; for others, it is something that brought them closer together.

Notions of the family and genetic relatedness were extremely significant in women's decisions to endure infertility treatment. Some could not move forward with donor eggs because they knew they could not accept a nongenetically linked child as their own. Many women wanted to be able to recognize themselves and their family members in the faces and behaviors of their children—to have other people around who are like themselves. This connects to the issues discussed earlier regarding kinship failures, especially in regard to inaccessible fathers. Infertility magnifies the sense of failure. For women experiencing infertility, the themes of not feeling connected—absent fathers, failed kinship, lack of genetic continuation, and failing as a woman—are recurrent.

Aging is a major reason why women decide to have a child on their own when they do. All except one woman in my study expressed the desire to have a child *with* a partner—whether female or male—rather than alone. These women described having gone through numerous relationships, whether with a man or a woman, and thus delaying their decision to have a child, hoping that the right relationship would come along. When it became apparent that "time was running out"—when they were in their late thirties—single women decided to have a child on their own. Lesbian couples attempting to conceive were also typically in their thirties. Both single women and lesbian couples delayed childbearing until they had completed their education or had gotten to stable points in their careers.

All of the women going through infertility emphasized the cost of treatment and their interactions with the medical system. They identified a major issue in the system that leads to excessive costs for infertility treatment among women without male partners: the ways in which infertility is diagnosed. For heterosexual couples, infertility is diagnosed after the couple has tried to conceive for a year or more. For women using donor sperm, thousands of dollars are spent before a diagnosis of infertility is ever conferred. These women all told me they wished they could have been granted an infertility work-up before ever starting the process of donor insemination so that they could either remedy the problem first or skip straight to the technology that would be most likely to get them pregnant and thus avoid spending thousands of dollars on "wasted sperm."

In the *Elusive Embryo*, Gay Becker (2000) describes the linkages between technology and culture and discusses how women and men experience their roles as consumers in the infertility industry and navigate the vast array of options available. Fertility practitioners choose some patients and reject others. Sometimes a patient may be rejected based on a practitioner's personal belief system regarding who is fit to procreate. Other times a prospective patient may be turned away because of her low odds of achieving a successful pregnancy, as a clinic's success rate is its bread and butter. Some fertility practitioners do continue to offer new options in order to achieve success, with increasing levels of medical management and cost: if home insemination does not work, then try IUI; if IUI does not work, then maybe GIFT or IVF, depending on the patient's resources; if her eggs are too old, then maybe donor eggs; and if her body cannot carry a pregnancy, then surrogacy is an option. Interestingly, as I conducted many of the interviews for Becker's work, starting in 1990 and ending in 2003, I noticed that heterosexual couples pursued the infertility treatment path far more extensively, and far more frequently, than the single women and lesbian couples I was interviewing for my research. Some of the heterosexual couples' exhaustive pursuit of fertility treatment options was due to a higher degree of encouragement from their physicians to try the next level of treatment.

Women's experiences with the medical community were varied. Some women had very positive experiences. Some saw medical professionals as insensitive to the issues of single women and lesbian couples—for example, many encountered the assumption that women were coming in to inseminate with their husbands' sperm. And some viewed medical practitioners as "monsters," technicians lacking any human qualities. But everyone in this research who pursued medical treatment for infertility viewed the underlying cultural and heteronormative assumptions of fertility care as an obstacle to getting quality care when they needed it and as contributing to wasted time and failure.

Some women who go through infertility treatment (approximately 30 percent) do eventually have a biological child. For the rest, infertility treatment is an exhausting, depressing, fruitless journey that appears to have no end in sight other than getting too old to pursue treatment with their own eggs. Women typically feel compelled to continue until they succeed, to keep trying new remedies or new technologies, always hoping that the next cycle will produce a pregnancy. Coming to terms with failure and deciding when to stop is probably one of the most difficult decisions to make. Many women become too emotionally or physically exhausted to continue. Most are afraid the infertility drugs will cause them to get cancer if taken too long. Many run out of money.

Across the globe, infertility comes with feelings of stigma and disempowerment (Inhorn 1995; Tremayne and Inhorn 2012). Infertile women in Egypt are often blamed for "reproductive failing and must bear the burden of overcoming it through a reproductive quest" (Inhorn 1994, 114). These feelings of stigma are equally true for women in the United States. When their efforts prove unsuccessful, many women—whether heterosexual, bisexual, lesbian, married, or single—engage in magical thinking and self-blame, believing that their infertility is caused by having mental blocks, not being open, bad Karma, promiscuity, former drug use, and so on. This is especially so when the cause of infertility is unexplained, but also even when there is clear evidence that the underlying cause may be a structural or hormonal problem with the body, such as polyps, a tipped uterus, or hormonal abnormalities. As Edward E. Evans-Pritchard ([1937] 1976, 22) describes in his classic book *Witchcraft, Oracles, and Magic among the Azande*, when a granary collapses and kills the people sitting underneath, the Azande recognize that bad things happen but ask, *Why* were those particular people sitting under that particular granary at that time? For them, the answer is witchcraft. People seek explanations to make meaning of their suffering. This was no less true for people seeking technological relief from infertility in the 1990s than it was for Azande seeking explanations for their grief in the 1930s.

The high cost of fertility treatment is also a reproductive justice issue (Shanley and Asch 2009). Social class, access to financial resources, and good health insurance that covers infertility treatment all determine which people can get the best possible care and have the best possible chances for reproductive success and which people cannot. Economic privilege is a determining factor in getting access to treatment, and people with access to resources can find a way to overcome the obstacles that would get in the way of their receiving care. Women in my study with more limited means, or no insurance, were forced to stop trying earlier, due to financial strain. Most of the women—indeed, most consumers in the infertility market—are marked by personal success. They are educated. They have good careers and make good money. They are used to taking on challenges and succeeding. Hence, "failure" to conceive a child is unthinkable. Women constantly asked themselves why conceiving a child is not like the rest of life's challenges, in which they have excelled.

As Charis Thompson states, "Involuntary childlessness is recognized as being one of the greatest forms of unhappiness and loss an adult woman might have to endure" (2005, 55). In their unrelenting quest for a biological child, patients become consumers and refuse to give up until they have exhausted all options, investing hope in the next level of technological options when the others have failed. Most women only stop when age puts them out of the running, as Marla described: "Infertility is gone. It's a dead issue with me now. It's because of my age, if nothing else. Yeah, the memory is still there, and the feeling I had for that brief moment I was pregnant will always be with me and I will always carry that loss. But now I need to close that chapter and try to focus on other things in my life." For Marla, and most other women who eventually stop without success, the decision to end treatment and "focus on other things" in life comes with sad relief.

8 · WHAT'S ALTERNATIVE ABOUT FAMILY?

> I think very early in parenting, in preschool, my daughter was quite aware of family constellations and the different kinds of families. It seemed to me, though, she had this longing to be like other families. I'm not sure it was about gender. It was more about having two parents.   —Sylvia, forty-three

> When I told my parents I was trying to get pregnant, they said, "Why would you do that? You're a lesbian."   —Rachel, thirty-five

In the 1990s, and even today, the word *alternative* was used to describe families that fall outside the heterosexual, married norm—especially two-mom families and two-dad families in which children are not the result of heterosexual procreation. When I first conceptualized this book, I used the term "alternative families" in the subtitle, but the term just did not sit right with me. A friend of mine had a similar problem with it and shared the book's original title with others in her Facebook network. Her friends, especially those in her LGBTQ community, expressed problems with the term: "Alternative to what?" "Alternative to whom?" "What about trans families?" and so on. I decided, instead, to borrow from Susan Golombok's (2015) *Modern Families* for the subtitle—a title inspired by the popular TV sitcom of the same name. This not only addresses the range of family-building and family structure options beyond the heteronormative nuclear family but also speaks to representations of family in current popular culture trends and how family is presented in television entertainment.

Anthropologists have had a long-standing interest in the study of kinship, including kinship system types (Morgan 1871), kinship networks and social processes in which blood relations are seen as the source of social cohesion (Radcliffe-Brown 1922), the role of kinship in maintaining the stability of institutions and communities (Malinowski 1922), and elementary forms of kinship and modes of exchange (Levi-Strauss [1949] 1969). The study of kinship is an analysis of what humans do with the "basic facts of life—mating, gestation, parenthood, socialization, siblingship, etc." (Fox 1967, 30).

David Schneider (1968, 1984) caused a shift in anthropological thinking about kinship by critiquing earlier notions that biogenetic ties formed the foundation of kinship universally across cultures. According to Schneider (1984), the idea that "blood is thicker than water," held by most Western anthropologists, was based more on their own ethnocentric positions than on cultural universals. His arguments were key in prompting new analyses that teased apart the biological and social elements of kinship, including how nurture may play more of a role in definitions of kin than blood ties (Holland 2012), as well as important critiques of how his view of kinship as a cultural system was based on heterosexual assumptions, which viewed heterosexual intercourse as a "means of establishing conjugality and procreativity" (Franklin 1997, 165).

Broadly defined, anthropologists think of kinship as a web of social relationships that may or may not have a biological connection. Drawing upon Schneider's work, Kath Weston further illuminated the complex meanings of kinship in the LGBTQ community, as many LGBTQ people forge new meanings of kinship beyond biological connection—particularly in response to rejection when disclosing a "stigmatized sexual identiy" (Weston 1995, 91). Additionally, feminist scholars have been instrumental in challenging the hegemony of the nuclear family (Thorne and Yalom 1982) and the bourgeois mythology of mother love as a biological given (Scheper-Hughes 1985).

Anthropological and feminist studies of kinship and the family are important when thinking about how donor-conceived families define themselves. Among female-partnered families, one of the mothers may actually have no genetic connection to the child while the other does, but they are both still considered mothers. A donor, who is a biological father, is not recognized as a social father. One's role as a parent is not necessarily rooted in genetic relatedness. Yet legal definitions of family do not necessarily reflect the day-to-day realities of people's lives, making families that do not adhere to heteronormative parameters particularly vulnerable.

The family is the fundamental unit in which children are socialized and learn values, norms, and behavior—more so than any other institution. Family structure has changed dramatically from the 1990s to today. Between the 1960s and 1990s, definitions of family broadened greatly. Family composition in the 1960s consisted primarily of a heterosexual, married couple and their children, and 73 percent of all children were living in a "traditional family" structure.

By the 1990s, definitions of family began to expand and include single parents, same-sex parent couples, grandparents parenting, blended families, and other arrangements. Yet mainstream American society remained uneasy about these shifting definitions of family, and often perceived families created outside the parameters of married heterosexual relationships as morally wrong (Brewer 2003; Doan, Loehr, and Miller 2014; Whitehead and Perry 2015, 2016). The traditional, nuclear family, consisting of a married man and woman and their biological children, was still held out as the moral imperative. Anything outside that was perceived as transgressing social, moral, and religious norms (Perry and Whitehead 2016). The presence of a father was seen as essential to a child's normal development. In 1999, an article published in *American Psychologist* was among the first to challenge that previously accepted claim, instead contending that successful parenting was not gender specific, that children do not necessarily need either fathers or mothers, and that any gender configuration of adults could parent well (Silverstein and Auerbach 1999).

According to a Pew Research Center report, as of 2014, fewer than half (46 percent) of U.S. kids under eighteen years of age are living in a home with two heterosexual, married parents in their first marriage, compared to 1980, when 61 percent lived in such a household (Livingston 2014). In 1980, 19 percent of children were living with an unmarried parent, while in 2014, 34 percent of children were. By the time a child reaches sixteen, almost half (46 percent) will live with a mother who is in a cohabiting relationship. While in the 1970s, 11 percent of all births were to unmarried women, by 2000 one-third of births were among unmarried women, including women with a partner but not married. The data do not account for children raised in same-sex partnered households, however, instead collapsing them into single-parent households. Data from the Williams Institute (Gates 2014) indicate that in 2013, 48 percent of lesbian-identified women and 20 percent of gay men were raising a child under age eighteen—including biological children, adopted children, and foster children. Among couples, 27 percent of female-partnered households include children under eighteen, compared to 11 percent of male-partnered couples (Gates 2014). Women are increasingly giving birth later and are also more likely to be college educated and in the workforce than before. In 2014, 40 percent of mothers were also primary wage earners (Livingston 2014). Many of these women-headed households are the result of divorce and men's abandoning their financial and parental responsibilities to their children.

In *The Origin of the Family, Private Property, and the State,* Friedrich Engels ([1884] 1972) addresses the rise of the nuclear family alongside increased awareness of the cause-and-effect relationship between sex and pregnancy and the production of a child. According to evolutionary theory, there was a perceived advantage for men to invest in their genetic heirs. Engels discusses this as leading a shift away from matrilineal and matrifocal societies toward patrilineal and patrifocal forms, with fathers at the head as providers and women as caretakers. Engels further states, "The first condition for the liberation of the wife is to bring the whole female sex back into public industry, and . . . this in turn demands that the characteristic of the monogamous family as the economic unit of society be abolished" (137–138). For Eleanor Burke Leacock (1972), the rise of the nuclear family was central to women's oppression, as well as to understanding the rise of capitalism and class society. Interestingly, Engels's predictions were coming to fruition, albeit almost a century later, but not always in the liberating way he imagined. Divorced, single women were at a serious economic disadvantage—especially when they attempted to maintain the nuclear family structure on their own rather than participate in more communal family arrangements.

The professional and financial gains some women have made have enabled them to take more control of their lives, including over decisions concerning when to have children, with whom to have children, and how they want to raise their children. In some ways, financial independence and technological advances can be seen as contributing to a rise in matrilineal, matrifocal families. Class and race, however, are crucial here. Carol Stack (1974), in *All Our Kin*, describes low-income urban black women who developed complex networks of real and fictive kin in order to find mutual support and strength in the face of poverty.

Most of the women in the present study developed networks for social and parental support, but the majority were from upper-middle-class white families, had college educations and advanced degrees, and were mostly professional women with the resources to support a child either on their own or with their female partners. Economic privilege plays an enormous role in women's reproductive autonomy and decisions surrounding family—especially through the use of technology.

This does not mean that single mothers and female-partnered couples with children do not experience parenting challenges, as do heterosexual couples. What is distinct, however, is that families that fall outside heteronormative standards are marginalized in ways that straight families are not. The women in my research all faced the standard difficulties and rewards of parenting, some on their own and some with their partner. The things that are unique to single-parent and female-partnered households include family reactions to the news of planned or impending motherhood, the everyday challenges of parenting, concerns regarding social acceptance or that kids will be stigmatized, decisions concerning when and how to tell a child he or she is donor conceived, managing children's feelings surrounding unknown donors, decisions regarding the role a known donor should have in a child's life, concerns about having one's family legally recognized, and so on. These are in addition to the universal concerns of how to raise healthy, well-adjusted children that all parents have.

Donor insemination and access to reproductive technologies enable women to choose parenting outside the confines of heterosexual relationships. As Kath Weston writes, "Insemination was the innovation many credited with motivating the lesbian baby boom, facilitating biological parenthood without requiring marriage, subterfuge, or heterosexual intercourse" ([1991] 1998, 169). The rise of sperm banks like The Sperm Bank of California and others that followed—which emerged with the specific intent to provide services to all women, regardless of marital status and sexual orientation—smoothed the path to motherhood for many. This was in direct opposition to the mainstream, heteronormative state, in which marriage was only permitted between a man and a woman, and children were to be the products of a heterosexual married union—an ideal that rapidly disintegrated amid rising divorce rates and reconfigured families.

Katrina Kimport's (2014) analysis of same-sex marriage in San Francisco in 2004—legal until the California Supreme Court subsequently voided it—addresses the linkages between heteronormativity, power, and the state, as well as how same-sex marriage is perceived as a direct affront to heterosexual privilege. Heterosexual privilege also entered into child custody cases. The courts reinforced a heteronormative requirement for the so-called best interests of the child by routinely denying lesbians custody of their children—whether conceived through donor insemination or in previous heterosexual relationships. For example, in one highly publicized case, Sharon Bottoms lost custody of her son to her mother, who had sued for custody on the grounds that her daughter's sexual orientation would damage the child's "psychological development," saying he would grow up confused about his sexual identity (Bull 1993, 24). The court granted custody to Bottoms' mother, with the judge stating that Sharon's lack of a high school education and signing of a movie contract about her life had influenced his decision against her (Lehr 1999, 5). In addition to lesbians losing custody to other family members, in female-partnered relationships, there were no legal protections for the nonbiological, nongestational mother, or for the rights of children to have access to both parents, since the maternal relationship was based on the biological connection to the child, rather than a social connection—a distinction that was not applied to heterosexual, married couples, as a child born in a marriage is presumed to be the child of both parents, regardless of biology. This resulted in a number of cases in which women who had entered into co-parenting with their partners lost all contact with the child or children upon separation.

Medical practices—especially infertility treatment—were the mechanisms through which mainstream prejudices controlled the reproduction of individual, nonconforming bodies, an example of what Michel Foucault (1980) refers to as "biopower." As mentioned in chapter 7, distinctions between "medical infertility" (inability to conceive after one year of trying through heterosexual sex) and "social infertility" (infertility arising from a lack of "natural access to sperm") provided an added barrier to same-sex couples and single women: while medical infertility was at least in part covered by insurance, social infertility was not. At the time, while some medical practitioners would provide access to donor sperm and fertility treatment for single women and lesbian couples, many would not. Even in the San Francisco Bay Area—which was liberal compared to the rest of the United States—women still faced obstacles to fertility care, with some medical practices acting as frontline enforcers of the discriminatory policies of the state. As Belinda, a forty-year-old single woman seeking treatment for infertility, told me in 1993,

> After almost a year of going through donor inseminations on my own through the sperm bank, I finally realized I was going to have to see a fertility specialist. My own doctor said I was going to need more specialized care than she could provide, so she gave me a list of names. I showed up at one doctor's office in San Francisco, and the receptionist starting asking me whether my husband was coming in so he could provide a sample. When I told her I wasn't married and I was using a donor, her response was, "Oh . . . Well, we can't help you here." I was shocked.
>
> There I was in a waiting room full of patients and they were turning me away because I wasn't married. I ran out of there. After that, I just kept calling office after office and asking them upfront if they would treat single women, so I wouldn't have to be humiliated like that again. I couldn't believe how many said no—in San Francisco! I finally found Dr. N., who was great, but I was shocked doctors would actually turn patients away.

Before the rise of sperm banks like The Sperm Bank of California—which emerged as sites of localized resistance to discriminatory medical practices— lesbians and gay men often entered into co-parenting or donor arrangements. MAIA Midwifery emerged as a hub for resources and connections for prospective LGBTQ parents, among other centers. However, the HIV/AIDS crisis dramatically reduced this method of family creation. Several women in this study first turned to a gay male friend to be a donor, only to find out when going through the medical testing that he was HIV positive or had had sex with an HIV-positive partner. One woman discovered that her donor was HIV positive after she had already conceived with him, and although she ended up fine, her entire pregnancy was fraught by a double trauma: the trauma of losing a dear friend to a horrible disease and the trauma of possibly being exposed to it herself. Sperm banks that offered services to all women—regardless of sexual orientation—offered a safer path to motherhood, with donors who were medically screened and sperm that was quarantined.

Rainbow Flag Health Services also provided new opportunities for men who had sex with men by reducing the potential risk of using donor sperm from this population and offering them pathways to relationships with children born from their sperm. Rainbow Flag not only helped women become mothers with donors they and their children could eventually meet but also enabled gay men to have genetic children and play a role beyond "donor" but not quite that of "father." It also provided an opportunity for people who preferred gay male donors, and provided fresh-sperm intrauterine insemination with known donors when no one else in Northern California would. The women to whom these children were born had the power to set the parameters of their child's relationship to their donor, as well as what kind of contact the donor would have with their child. Sperm banks contributed to the emergence of new definitions of family and reframed biological and social relationship categories.

While technologies and informal arrangements gave rise to an array of family forms, even in the face of changing family structures, challenges remained. By conventional thinking, it was assumed that if a woman was lesbian, she either did not want to have a child or was not entitled to be a mother. Having a child as a single woman continued to be stigmatized in mainstream society. Men having children in donor father arrangements also struggled to have their roles recognized. Deciding to have a child outside a married, heterosexual relationship also forced conversations some did not feel prepared to have.

I'M HAVING A BABY

For single women and lesbian couples who wanted to have a child through donor insemination, starting that process often involved telling people—friends or family—about their plans to conceive a child. Disclosing this news to others was not without risk. Due to social stigma attached to either their sexuality or their decision to become a single parent, many women faced judgment and scorn instead of the congratulatory messages a married, straight woman would receive when announcing such news. Heterosexual couples usually share the news of a pregnancy after it has already occurred. Women without male partners often share their decision to try to have a child before they ever conceive. Thus, this decision is shared earlier and is more public than it is for straight couples—which makes them vulnerable to scrutiny.

Jocelyn was forty by the time she realized she wanted to have a child. Having been raised in an abusive family, she had feared she would not make a good mother. She was more anxious about telling her parents she conceived with a donor after leaving her husband of fourteen years.

> People talk about biological clocks, but for me that wasn't really it. I had never wanted a child before because I was afraid I would be abusive, like my parents. Finally, in therapy, I reached the point where I realized I had a choice not to pass that down and that I really wanted to have a child.
>
> And the next decision I had to make was whether to stay in the fourteen-year relationship I was in. He had a vasectomy a long time ago, and he was also abusive, verbally, plus he had his own kids and didn't want more. So I decided to get divorced. I couldn't sleep at night. He would yell at me right at bedtime and I would chew my fingernails all night. But in thinking about leaving I started getting a deeper passion to have a baby—just not with him.
>
> So I moved out, got my own house, changed jobs, quit drinking, and started taking prenatal vitamins to prepare my body to get pregnant with a donor. After just three months of inseminations, I got pregnant.

I told my brother I was pregnant, but I asked him not to tell our mom and dad. For some reason he thought this baby would "bring our family together," since our parents were divorced and not really speaking to each other.

But I dreaded telling my parents. For them, not being married and having a child was worse than being married and having a child in an abusive household. When I finally told my dad he was appalled. He literally blew up and said, "I won't be around her." After Bea was born, I sent him pictures of the baby. His only response was, "Photos received. Good luck. Dad." Typical for him—abuse through withdrawal and neglect.

The nicest thing my mother said to me when I told her I was pregnant was, "I don't think potato chips are good for the baby." For a lot of women that kind of comment would really annoy them, but I kind of liked it because it implied that she did care.

After the baby was born, I waited a couple of weeks before I called her to invite her down to see the baby. She said she couldn't make it because she had to "wash the dog." So yeah, my dad is indifferent, and my mom is just mean. I finally told her not to call me anymore.

Jocelyn's experience points to the fear and obstacles some women face when trying to have a child outside heterosexual procreative expectations. At the age of forty, she did not have the luxury of time to wait for the "right relationship" to come along. Rather than expressing joy at having a grandchild, her parents focused on the stigma of having a child out of wedlock. Rather than bringing the family together, as Jocelyn's brother had hoped, her decision to have a child without a husband drove an even deeper wedge. She eventually hired an attorney to draft a legal package that included a financial power of attorney and a medical power of attorney in order to protect both herself and her baby from her mother and ensure her daughter would never spend a moment alone with her.

Tara, thirty-five, had a vastly different experience from Jocelyn's. Tara defined herself as bisexual and polyamorous. She used a donor with whom she had a sexual relationship while trying to conceive, with an agreement that they would stop sleeping together as soon as she got pregnant. She explained her experience of telling friends and family about her pregnancy:

My mom is very traditional in a nontraditional sense. I had been telling her for years that I wanted to have a baby on my own, and she kept saying, "Just wait. You should hang in there until you meet somebody nice." Most moms tell their kids to wait until they find a nice man and settle down, but my mom kept saying, "Someday you'll meet a nice woman and settle down." She wants me to be a lesbian. She wasn't keen on me being bisexual at all. She was like, "Men are not to be trusted. They don't stick around. You should meet a nice woman instead, and then have a baby."

So coming out about my sexuality to my parents was never a problem. But Ken, my donor, didn't want to tell anyone about the pregnancy right away, and for me keeping secrets is really hard. And it was especially difficult with my friend, and sometimes lover, Jenna. She and I weren't romantically involved at the time, but the three of us were like the Three Musketeers, so we had to tell her because we couldn't keep it a secret from her. So pretty soon, we both ended up telling everyone.

So yeah, everyone knows. My whole family has met Ken. And Jenna tells everyone she's the father, and they're both going to be there for the delivery. The hardest part, though, is my lesbian friends. Everyone would be fine with me being a lesbian and having a child, but being bisexual and using natural methods of conception gets a lot of negative responses.

I mean, people ask me who my turkey-baster donor is and when I tell them I actually conceived the old-fashioned way, they're like, "You mean you had sex with a man?" And when I tell them I'm bisexual and I do it all the time, they really don't get it. And then they say, "Donor? He can't be a donor unless there's a turkey baster involved." Who says I can't have sex with a man to get pregnant and he's my donor? So I stick to dating bisexual women and bisexual men, and then I don't have to explain myself as much.

Telling her family about her decision to have a child was mostly a positive experience for Tara, unlike Jocelyn. Her mother wanted her to have a child in the context of a relationship so she would have the support of a partner and the child would have two loving parents, regardless of sexual orientation. For Tara, "coming out" about her decision to have a child, and about her sexuality, left her open to criticism in her social circles among her lesbian friends.

You know, everyone wants to put you in this category: "Are you lesbian or are you straight? Are you co-parenting with your donor or with your girlfriend?" And on and on. And I just don't fit into these boxes. Just because I have a girlfriend right now, doesn't mean she and I are co-parenting—we're not ready for that step. I decided to have this baby right now on my own. And it's a huge sigh of relief because now I'm not sitting here thinking, "Am I having a baby with you? Or you? Or you?" Man or woman. I'm not going to hook up with someone just so I can have this baby. I do believe that it takes a village to raise a child, and I wouldn't be doing this without the support of my sister and mother and father and girlfriend and my best friend and all of these wonderful people in my life.

Tara's relationship with her known donor is also unconventional. If a woman has a child through sexual intercourse with a man—even if they have a written legal agreement stating he is a donor and not a father—by law he is still considered the father. By having a brief sexual relationship with Ken, she placed an enormous amount of trust in him that he would not contest their legal agreement and seek paternal rights. This was balanced by his trust in her. She relinquished rights to child support in their legal agreement, but if she changed her mind, the courts would force him to pay support.

Lesbians who seek motherhood often face a double challenge: coming out about their sexual orientation and about the decision to mother while lesbian. Women who already had disclosed their sexual orientation to their families and friends confronted assumptions that motherhood would be out of the question, as if being a lesbian and a mother were mutually exclusive (Lewin 1981; Lewin and Lyons 1982; Mamo 2007). For example, Rachel explained her parents' reaction when she told them she was looking for a sperm donor: "I had finally made the decision to do this and I wanted to share it with my parents, because I wanted them to know they could be grandparents. Their response was, 'Why would you do that? You're a lesbian.' It really stung, you know. I thought they had gotten over that and then I realized they were never going to get it. They would never really understand or accept me. I mean, just because I'm attracted to women doesn't mean I don't want to have a child."

Others have to navigate a complicated terrain when disclosing their status as both mother and lesbian—especially when they have not previously come out to family members. For example, Bonnie and Sharon, whom I first interviewed in 1992 and then later in 1997, explained how telling Bonnie's parents they were trying to conceive a child added complications and stress to an already strained relationship. In 1992, Sharon had still not told her father that her relationship with Bonnie was a romantic one:

BONNIE: God, I came out about eight or nine years ago and my mother reacted very badly and she's still reacting fairly badly. She finally realizes that Sharon is here to stay, but we're not even allowed to touch in front of her. We can't talk about anything or any of our friends. Anything that has to do with being a lesbian—which is part of who I am—I can't talk about. When I first came out she didn't call me for about six or seven months.

SHARON: I think her mom has gotten better over the last nine years, but the whole baby thing was a major setback. She had a hard enough time wrapping her head around the idea that her daughter had a lesbian lover, but now that her daughter and her lover are making babies, she just can't seem to comprehend the how and why of it.

But my brothers have been great! One brother and his wife are going through infertility treatment, so we talk all the time and they've been really supportive. My father still doesn't even know we're lovers, though—and we've been together forever.

DIANE: What does he think, then, if he doesn't know you're in a relationship? How do you hide that?

SHARON: Well, I'm not very close to my dad, so it isn't that difficult because we're not around him that much. But he just thinks Bonnie is my best friend.

BONNIE: Yeah, but her brothers are better than anyone could ever hope for. Aside from them, we can't really count on anybody except friends. We sort of have to make our own family.

Lack of parental support among some lesbians choosing motherhood leads them to rely more on their friends or social networks—"the families they choose," as Weston puts it ([1991] 1998)—rather than the families in which they were raised. Some lesbians hide their sexuality from some or all of their family members. But the limitations on what one does or does not choose to disclose affect the ability to be oneself around the people who are supposed to love one unconditionally. I learned in 1997 that Sharon had not disclosed her relationship to her father until after Bonnie delivered their first child in 1993. The relationship with each of their respective parents continued to be strained throughout the birth of their first child, and it was only beginning to improve after Sharon delivered their second child prematurely:

BONNIE: We had a really bad experience when we had my mom here when I was delivering Andrea. I really didn't want her there in the delivery room, and she kept going in and out of the delivery room. And at some point Sharon told her she could wait in the waiting room and she'd call her when I was about to deliver.

SHARON: I think she felt left out.

BONNIE: Well, she just left the hospital. Left. I found out later she decided to have Thanksgiving with her friends down in Los Angeles. When she called she was really cold. I was pretty upset. You don't walk out when your daughter is having a baby and then call a half hour later and lay down some guilt trip because I'm not paying enough attention to her!

So when Sharon went into premature labor, I didn't even want her here. I didn't want that constant reminder of my mom ruining our birth—especially because it was really high risk. And then when I called her to tell her our son was in the NICU [neonatal intensive care unit], and about how stressful it was, she never asked me how I was, or how Sharon was. She just said, "Well, he's not *really* your son." She just had to get that jab in.

Bonnie and Sharon perceived Bonnie's mother's behavior as being due to her inability to full accept their relationship. Although they both say their respective families are coming around and their parents are actively involved as grandparents, the feeling of not being accepted because of their sexual orientation remains. Both Bonnie and Sharon felt that their respective parents would have been far more supportive if they were having children in heterosexual relationships.

Sperm donors can have similar challenges telling their families about both a child conceived from their donations and their sexuality—especially those who want to be known and have a relationship with the child. Robert, a Rainbow Flag donor introduced in chapter 4, told me about his experiences both when he initially came out as gay to his family and when he told them he had a child from sperm donation:

So my dad is really hard-core Catholic. When I told him I was gay he did not take it well, and pretty much refused to speak to me. My mom was kind of caught in the middle because we had this really authoritarian household and he treated her as if she was one of his children. . . .

One day I got this call from Leland. It was like two years after I donated, and I kind of wondered whatever came of that. And he said, "Congratulations, you're in the gene pool. The mother should be contacting you in about three months." And then I got a letter from her soon after that. It was really exciting! So, of course, I wanted to tell my family that I had a kid out there and we'd be able to meet him and his mother, but I really struggled with it.

So I went and met Ingrid, the mother, for the first time and her baby, and started getting to know them. She and her partner talked about wanting the baby to have this extended family, which for me was great, and also have me involved in his life. When I told my family, my mom and brothers were fine, but my dad absolutely refused to see him or his mothers or have any of them in his house. His response was, "That's immoral and unethical and I want nothing to do with it," and walked away. That's the only thing, and the last thing, he said to me.

I wanted everyone to meet Ingrid and her son over Christmas, and my dad absolutely refused. My mom has gone over to Ingrid's with me to meet them, but my dad . . . And the real irony is my brother had a kid out of wedlock from a one-night stand. And he accepts my brother's son without any problem and talks all the time about his grandson, but he doesn't even want to acknowledge that my son exists. It's not fair to my son. He's just a baby.

My mother has since said that she had talked with him and he said that he would be willing to meet the child but not the mother. And I said, "Pop, package deal."

So with his mom and her girlfriend, on the other hand, it's getting pretty familial. I went over to their house Christmas morning and then went to my parents' house Christmas dinner. But because of the situation my father has put me in, if this continues, my first priority will be to the mother and child, because that's where my priority belongs, to my new family.

At the same time, though, I want to respect Ingrid's boundaries because she told me that one of the hardest things about choosing a donor who would be known was that she was terrified he would file for custody of her son. And that would be the saddest thing I could think of is that a mother could lose her child. So it's a fine line I walk all the way around.

Robert's story reveals a range of concerns people face when forming families in ways that defy conventions. First is the issue of explaining to those close to you the decision to have a child either alone or in a same-sex relationship. Second, if family members already struggle with accepting one's sexual orientation, they are even more likely to reject the idea that one should bring children into same-sex family environments. Third, many people who cannot find acceptance within their families of origin find themselves creating new families or support systems with people who share their values and views. Fourth, creating families through these technologies and alternative arrangements expands traditional definitions of family for a child—mother with no father, two mothers, two fathers, donors, and hybrid donor fathers. Those who cling to tradition often perceive these families as dangerous because they defy prescribed social roles and "natural categories," as has been addressed by anthropologist Mary Douglas (1970).

DAY-TO-DAY FAMILY LIFE

Carolyn and I had many conversations over several years while I was doing this fieldwork, often meeting at a Berkeley café. Already a single mother of two teenage daughters from a former relationship, she decided to have a third child through donor insemination at thirty-five, before her "time ran out." For Carolyn, the challenge was not telling people she was pregnant but rather telling them how she conceived. She worried about how that would reflect on her and whether she would be taken seriously as a graduate student. She recounted,

> My experience is really different with this pregnancy, with a donor, compared to when I had my other daughters while in a relationship with their father. Before, I really wanted to do things the "right way." But now, that's not important to me. I just want to have another child. And there's this whole question about feeling deserving and undeserving—like if you choose to be a single mother you've lost your right to complain, or feel lonely at times, or ask for support.
>
> And people who don't know you make assumptions and call you "Mrs.," and are happy for you and people who do know you make assumptions and react with sympathy, as if it were an accident.
>
> I had dinner with my adviser a few weeks ago and now that I'm obviously pregnant, she asked me about it. She kind of touched my hand and said, "Well, just look at it as a gift." And I thought about telling her, "No. This was my decision and I got pregnant on purpose." But I couldn't do it. If I told her that, I knew I would suddenly be seen as not being a serious, committed student. You don't get sympathy or support when you've made a conscious decision. And that's really difficult because when you're a single parent, you need support regardless.
>
> And, you know, there's a lot of talk about this Single Mothers by Choice group, but I kind of have a problem with that. I think when we emphasize that we're

single or married or whatever, we're driving wedges between women in different situations. A lot of married women are really single as far as I can see and a lot of single mothers have men and other people in their lives that provide a lot of support.

Then there are people I thought would be really supportive—some of my closest friends—and they think it's really weird I'm doing this and have a lot of trouble with it, especially the married ones. One friend, who is in a miserable marriage, keeps saying, "How are you going to raise your son without a father? Look at the statistics on single parents." And there's all this judgment that it's better to be miserable and raise a child in a bad marriage than alone. So you kind of start re-evaluating your friendships in this process because—especially as a single mom—you need to be around supportive people.

Carolyn's experience demonstrates not only how different circumstances surrounding conception and parenting alone are perceived but also how perceptions directly affect social support. Single, straight women who conceive with intent are considered responsible for creating their own difficult situation, and they may be judged more harshly for using a donor than they would be if they had a one-night stand in a bar and accidentally conceived. The prevailing perspective that it is better to have a child in a dysfunctional marital relationship than alone because "children need a father" leads many single mothers like Jocelyn and Carolyn to forge new friendships and let less supportive friends drift away.

Jocelyn, who had been married for fourteen years and raised two stepchildren from the ages of four and six, had seen both the challenges of parenting with someone and as a single woman.

When you're married and raising kids, yeah, you have someone who maybe will go to the store on their way home from work, maybe will help bathe the kids and put them to bed, do homework, help financially, and all those things. But at the same time, you're counting on them to do that stuff and you're resenting them when they don't. And my ex and I, sometimes we would get into fights about child-rearing and who was going to do what. But other times were really nice, especially before he started getting abusive, and we would do things together as a family.

I don't think single women have more stuff to deal with, just different stuff.

And there's statistics that show that single women have it easier the first year because they don't have to deal with a husband, and all of the demands a relationship can put on you. But still, practical things can have an impact, especially when you're tired. They say to never leave the baby alone in the house. Okay, great, now you've got to take the trash cans out to the street. And the bin of newspapers that's too heavy for you to lift, so you put her in the backpack and take her out to do those chores. So I'm not going to get angry if someone else doesn't do what they say they're going to do, or do their part. I know I have to do it all on my own.

And yeah, of course I'd love to have a mate. But not any mate. I'm not interested in the wrong guy. When I was married, I was lonely. I'm less lonely now that
I'm alone and raising my daughter.

While Jocelyn did express feelings of loneliness and sometimes wished she had
a partner, for her, having a child on her own was vastly preferable to having a child
in an abusive marital relationship. Jocelyn's career success had afforded her the
ability to buy her own home after her divorce. She did not need her husband for
financial support, or even for emotional or logistical support. For her, having a
mate was not a requirement for having a child.

The notion that all children need two parents—a mother and a father—in
order to be exposed to the proper role models and gendered standards of behavior for boys and girls is based on a romanticized notion of the "traditional
family"—a family form that has been on the decline since the 1960s. This perspective not only denies the fact that same-sex or single-headed households can and
do provide stable, healthy environments in which to raise children but also glosses
over the fact that some heterosexual, two-parent household are not particularly
well adjusted or healthy. Many women I spoke to repeated a similar thought: Why
do women who have children without a male partner endure so much stigma and
scrutiny when there are so many children raised by abusive, drug-addicted, alcoholic parents who are heterosexual and married? These women believe that the
priority should be a stable home with a loving parent (or parents), rather than what
they perceive as an outdated and restrictive standard.

KNOWN DONORS, DONOR UNCLES, AND DONOR DADS

Whereas Carolyn and Jocelyn both used anonymous donors and parented primarily alone, Deena's decision to use a known donor provided her both with
parental autonomy as the sole legal and custodial parent and with regular support. Her donor, Babak, has an ongoing relationship with his biological child,
having a role "like an uncle," according to Deena. This arrangement offers their
son the opportunity to have a relationship with his donor father without Deena
having to worry about her own autonomy and authority as a single parent. For
Deena and Babak, this family structure has been working well. As Deena related,
"For me, this has been like the best of both worlds. I still have all rights and
responsibilities, and questions like if I decide to move or something aren't an
issue. He's my son. But Babak has been here and very supportive. He's very
involved now. He's been like an uncle, I think—and a friend. He comes over
twice a week and makes me dinner and takes him out for walks, which my brother
does too." I talked to Babak separately, to find out his perspective on being a
known donor, his friendship with Deena, and his relationship with his biological
child.

BABAK: I had always thought in the back of my mind that maybe I'd want to have a child someday, but I just pushed that down once I came out. And then Deena and I started talking about wanting to have a child after she broke up with her girlfriend. I thought about it a lot and I had some other friends—a gay man and his friend who was lesbian—who were co-parenting like this, and their daughter was twelve and everyone was really happy, so I thought, "Why not?"

At first, I thought I would be happy with photos and maybe flying out once a year, but then the more I started thinking about it the more I realized I wanted to be more involved than that. So I moved to California.

Once I moved out and Deena got pregnant, she introduced me to a friend of hers, Lida, who was forty and straight and really wanted to have a kid. So I did it for her, too. With her it was more formal though. She put me through a pretty strict interview.

And we all have our contracts, but the contract is very harsh in that it says that I have no rights or responsibilities. So it protects me but it also doesn't allow any leeway. I mean, it even says that this contract is enforceable regardless of what relationship develops between the donor and the child. And so that felt very hard, but luckily things have developed very differently.

DIANE: So what kind of contact do you have with the kids?

BABAK: With Deena, I come over a couple times a week and make dinner, or take Samuel out to the park and things like that. He's still too young for me to take him overnight, but hopefully someday I'll be able to. But I have a key to Deena's house and can pretty much come by any time. With Lida, it took her longer to trust me, but she's not as social as Deena is and she has fewer child care people in her community. So the trump card I have is that I'm available to babysit any time.

DIANE: What do the kids call you?

BABAK: Candace, Lida's daughter, calls me "Baba" and Sam calls me "daddy." And Deena thinks of me as an uncle, like her brother, which I guess is OK. But it's really up to the kids as to what they want to call me. But Deena and I are working on a second child right now, so I guess it's working out OK.

And it's kind of funny. Just today, right before you came over, I got a call from Lida and she was talking to me about setting up for a breakfast over the weekend and I said, "Who are you inviting?" And she said, "Just you, and Deena, and Sam. Just the family." That was the first time she referred to me as family and it's been three years now. So that was nice.

DIANE: When you first thought about being a known donor, did you have any concerns?

BABAK: I think my main issue was the fear around whether I would have enough contact with the children. I was afraid of what some of my family would think. My father's family, who are Anglo-Americans, I'm out to. I was afraid what they would think of having to go through the issue of accepting me as gay and having to deal with this issue. But they're just thrilled and supportive because everyone is happy when you have children. Now, my mother's family is Muslim, originally from Pakistan, and I'm not really out to them. I mean, I just told them that I had done this, that I had children with two women, and that I wasn't living with the women at all. That was perfectly normal. I mean, they're Pakistani but living in the Caribbean. They were just thrilled to know that I had children and that I was in touch with them.

Deena, Lida, and Babak, and the children born from these arrangements, push the boundaries of what we normally define as family. Although Babak is biologically a father, socially he is father, honorary uncle, and donor, shifting between these categories depending on the situation and with whom he is interacting. While he is "family," he is in some ways a marginalized member whose involvement with his biological children and their respective mothers is vulnerable. Lida and Deena are both undeniably mothers, and they maintain control over the level of involvement their respective children have with their biological father. On the one hand, Babak provides both women with support, their children have contact with him, and Babak has a relationship with children he might otherwise not have had. However, his role within the family could potentially be threatened if he pushed for more contact or more responsibility. Aware of this delicate balance, Babak knows he has to navigate the appropriate amount of contact by offering to babysit without claiming full paternity. This idea of men "babysitting" their children, however, can also be found among straight, married dads. In Babak's case, it is the mothers who have full parental rights—unless he wants to pursue a paternity claim in court.

Female-headed families with children conceived though insemination by a known donor add a new twist to anthropological studies of kinship. Men who provide sperm have a range of roles on the paternity spectrum. Anonymous sperm bank donors normally have no contact with their biological children, but some may actually meet them once the child is legally an adult. Robert was an exception to that rule and became involved in the child's life from early infancy, with no prior relationship to the child's mothers. Babak decided a long-distance relationship with his donor-conceived children was not sufficient and opted to be as involved as his children's respective mothers would permit, while still respecting the mothers' relationships as sole custodial and legal parents. Ethan, a forty-one-year-old known donor to a lesbian couple with a newborn infant, summed it up this way:

On the one hand, you have donors who make their deposits, get paid, and have total noninvolvement. They're biological fathers, but they're not real fathers. On the other hand, you have your live-in dads who are raising kids, giving the baby the bottle at three o'clock in the morning, and super involved. Somewhere in the middle, you've got your very traditional husbands who do nothing, or are detached, or divorced absentee fathers. Then you have your gay dads who are not there as full-time co-parents, but often they're more involved than straight dads who don't have custody.

For me, this is my child, my daughter, but still not. It's not the same thing as being married and fully raising a child, and it's also different than my relationship with my partner's daughter, because she and I don't have that biological connection. And I understand the mothers want to be in control. It's their child, their family, and I'm OK with that. And, because I'm gay, I never, ever envisioned myself as the head of the family, or a father. In this way, the moms include me. I get to be a part-time, involved dad—which is all I really want anyway—and they get to have the say in how they raise their daughter. I now have a different model and a whole different sense of what being a gay man and a father might mean.

Sean and Ethan had been together for eleven years when I first met them in their San Francisco, Noe Valley, Victorian flat in the summer of 2000. Ethan greeted me at the door, while Sean was not yet home from work. I walked in and noticed the telltale signs of a young girl's presence—several baskets of neatly organized toys, a small pink jacket hanging in the entryway, a pair of girls' sneakers underneath, a book bag, and other items. Sean was a known donor dad to a seven-year-old daughter, Sara, who spent about 25 percent of her time with Sean and about 75 percent of her time with her mothers. Ethan was also a known donor to a three-week-old daughter named Chloe, with Marlene and her partner, Robin. Robin also has another daughter, whom she adopted before she met Marlene, and they raise the child together. Sean and Ethan moved to Noe Valley from the Castro in 1993, shortly before Sean's daughter was born, so they could be in the same neighborhood as the mothers, as well as in a neighborhood they saw as more family friendly.

I talked to Ethan and Sean separately and together. In many ways, their family structure demonstrates how many gays and lesbians were creating families before the HIV/AIDS crisis and the rise of the sperm-banking industry. Although less common after the rise of HIV, some women still perceived the advantages of having children with someone who would be known to the child—and to them—rather than with a complete stranger whom they most likely would never meet. This desire among some women to have a known donor opened up opportunities for gay men to parent that they otherwise may not have had. Sean explained to me what he sees as a recurring theme discussed in his gay dads' group:

One of the issues is the dads not having enough of a voice. From a psychological standpoint, there's a hesitation for the men to say, "This is what I want." They're kind of like waiting in the sidelines to be given something, or waiting and taking their cues from what's happening from the mothers.

It's kind of like an imbalance. It's OK for the moms to be late bringing the kids to meet up with us, but it's a horribly intolerable thing if we're ever late to meet up with the moms. If I'm late, "What have you done with my child?" Or "You simply can't be trusted, can you?" So it's almost like the moms become our moms. It's a dynamic I've seen among straight couples too, with or without children. So it's a bit controlling, but at the same time, we know the kids are well cared for, and the moms have it all wired, and that's good for the kids.

But it's difficult, because you kind of have to hang back and wait for them [the moms] to invite you in. So with Chloe, her mom and I agreed early on I would be able to have her 25 percent of the time. But then the baby comes, and that doesn't really happen. You know, they're nursing. So it's like, "OK, when are you going to be done nursing?" And it's another six months, or six more months, and the child is two. At some point the mother just has to learn to trust that the baby is going to be OK, and that the dad is going to be capable of feeding and changing diapers, and that's a good thing. Figure out how to include him. And the guy, the donor, he can contribute by figuring out what's going to help the mom—you know go out and buy her a pastrami sandwich, help her, be consistent. Then everyone is more relaxed and happy.

And it's weird, in a lot of ways it's the typical conflicts that happen between men and women when it comes to child-rearing but, you know, you're both gay, and in these other relationships and households, and trying to make it all work because you all love this baby that you created together. And then sometimes, the other, nonbiological mother might feel like you're taking over her role as the child's other parent. So you have to balance it all. It's traditional and not traditional all at the same time. But really, I think there's something intrinsically different about being a mother and being a father. For mothers, the child comes out of your body. Many women have this really overwhelming need to have children. Even in my gay dads' group, I don't see men having this driving need to have a child. It's nice when it happens but it's not overwhelming.

Ethan, a new father, explained to me how he first decided to be a known donor for Marlene within the context of his relationship with Sean:

Sean and I had been together for a couple of years, and we were part of this group of friends. This was about 1989, and two of his closest friends both died of AIDS, and we are all part of this group that provided emotional support. Jean was a part of that group and she approached Sean and asked him if he would be a donor for her. Before that, neither one of us had ever thought we'd ever be parents. So he and I were talking to Jean a lot, and talking to each other, about what that might look like for Sean to have a child with her. That was what first made me realize that this was something I could do.

So after Sara was born, I started thinking about it too. Then last year, Marlene approached me and asked if I'd consider being a donor for her. Sean and I talked a lot about what it meant for him to be a dad. I've been around his daughter a lot, but it's not like he and I are raising her together, and he really encouraged me to do this.

So when the opportunity came to be a donor for Marlene, I think I was much more ready to think about a more active role for myself, and really how much better it would be to be a dad with a child in the vicinity, in the neighborhood actually. Secondly for me I would say was a sense of being able to do something to help another person. And then moving from there to a sense of how wonderful it would be to actually have a role and participate myself. I'm part of a gay dads' group and I think for many of the guys in that group, I think their own desire to be a father came before their interest in helping a woman fulfill her wish. I think for me it went in the opposite order. I wanted to help her first, and then realized this was a great opportunity for me to be a dad too.

Marlene said they wanted to have somebody who at least would be known and would be open to having some involvement, but they didn't want a full co-parent. And that was pretty much what I was looking for. So I told them I would do this, but I wanted to be involved and I wanted to be called "dad"—not an uncle or something—because that's what I would be. Her dad.

I think it's so much more sensible if women, if lesbians are looking to become mothers to have a known donor, to include a man. I do think it's good for a child to have someone to call dad. I know for a lot of women being a mother means taking control, but there's a . . . I just think it's healthier. I guess it's my own male prejudice. And I think that's the neat thing that gay men and lesbians are coming together jointly to raise children.

Sean echoed that perspective in his description of his own experience:

At first, I thought I could kind of just be a donor and I guess I could be known as the uncle. And then I started thinking about it more and talking about it more. And I came to the conclusion that I really . . . I couldn't do it that way. If I was going to do it, I wanted to be a dad. And maybe being the dad would mean something entirely different from what people thought of as the dad. But I still would be the dad, you know. We'll re-create what that means.

So after Sara was born, I actually started by having a diaper fund. I said, "You know what? I'll give you diaper service." I was going to give Tracy it as a gift for six months and then I just started paying for the diapers forever. And then when she didn't need diapers I said, "You know, why don't I just give you this money every month." It seems to be a nice amount. And then it grew a little bit, and now I'm basically agreeing to pay 25 percent for education. So, I'm paying 25 percent of the tuition.

And it's incredible. I mean, I just feel incredibly blessed and incredibly lucky to have this wonderful little girl that calls me daddy, and she's so clever and bright and fun.

Throughout the stories of known donor dads, there is a recurrent theme regarding what it means to be a father in the absence of full parental rights. Donor dads address the delicate balance of creating a comfortable relationship with the mothers of their children, and not pushing for more contact than the mothers—the legal parents—are comfortable with, in order to have a relationship with their child. While in some ways they are building new models of what it means to be a father—especially a gay father—at the same time there is something traditional about these arrangements. The mothers have primary caretaking responsibilities. They make the main decisions concerning the day-to-day care of children and where they go to school, their activities, and so on. They invite the donors to participate to the degree to which they are comfortable, while the donor dads are concerned about not crossing a line that could interfere with their relationship with their child. In some ways, this is a very conventional dynamic found in many heterosexual families.

In the interviews with women who used known donors—whether straight, bisexual, or lesbian, single or part of a couple—all expressed a desire to have decision-making power and to be in control of the relationship between donor and child. For many, this need for control stemmed from a fear that someone could take their child. Straight, married mothers also often face the fear of losing custody of their children in the event of a divorce. However, for lesbian mothers, this fear was connected, in part, to their marginalized status as mothers outside the realm of heteronormative social conventions. For women who used known donors, though, the need for control was offset by a sense that they did not want their children to wonder where they came from, or that it was important for a child to have some kind of relationship with a biological father. To have a gay man as a donor was seen as a safer option than using a straight man, however, since it would be difficult for a gay men to argue that a lesbian would be an unfit mother due to her sexual orientation.

For women who used anonymous sperm bank donors, the need for control over custody was accompanied by a fear that their custody could be challenged. This was especially true in lesbian families that prioritized a nuclear family model in which to raise their children, without interference from a third-party donor. In all fairness, the fear of losing custody is not unfounded. Lesbian couples were not able to have their relationships legally recognized, and many who had children in former relationships lost custody of their children because of their sexual orientation. Single mothers who had children in relationships were also vulnerable. Having a child with a donor—especially an anonymous donor—meant they would not have to worry about their child being taken away from them. Some lesbian couples also turned to the courts in order to have the parental rights of the nongenetic mother legally recognized, so that her relationship to the child would be legally protected.

WHO'S MY DONOR DADDY?

Most single women and lesbian couples using a sperm donor plan to tell their children how they were conceived and provide whatever information they can about their donor. For this reason, women using a sperm bank donor prefer to find someone who has agreed to have his identity released when the child turns eighteen, if not sooner. This factors into how women choose donors in the first place, as discussed in chapter 5. Not only do women want what is often called "identity-release" sperm, but they also want to make sure they choose a donor whose profile speaks to them, who sounds like someone they would like as a person, and whose profile contains positive traits they can be proud of when sharing that information with their child, as most are inclined to do.

Sabrina is a single, lesbian mother who started thinking about trying to conceive on her own when she was thirty-five. She had first planned on using a known donor who was gay and a close friend of hers. Shortly before she was about to start inseminating, he—like so many gay men in the 1990s—discovered he was HIV positive. Like other women who considered using known, gay donors, Sabrina not only had to choose someone else but also had to face losing a dear friend she wanted to co-parent with. She had another gay friend who agreed to be her donor, but after four or five unsuccessful attempts, they gave up trying. "I was pretty despondent," Sabrina told me. "I wasn't planning on going the sperm bank route because I wanted my child to know who her biological father is."

In order to have at least a partially known donor, she decided to try Rainbow Flag Health Services and went to one of their Egg Meets Sperm networking mixers to meet a prospective donor.

There we were. Women on one side of the room, and men on the other. It felt really weird—like every terrible thing about prom. It was like a popularity contest, and we were all scouting each other out according to looks, personality, economics. So here we were at this champagne brunch and we're supposed to be having babies together. It was absurd.

So after I left there I decided I was just going to have to go the sperm bank route. And I felt the most important thing in reading this donor profile was that some day my child was going to read it too. So I wanted someone who ethically felt right and someone who was mature, who thought this out, who would be willing to meet the children, and who didn't just say, "I'm doing this for the money." How can you tell your child their donor—their genetic father—just needed money? You know?

So he wrote this beautiful essay about what it means to him to be a father and how he wanted more kids, but his wife didn't, so he wanted to be able to help other people have kids. So, when I read that in his profile I felt like, "OK, he sounds like a nice, altruistic kind of guy and I can hand this to my child." And even if she's terribly upset about having a donor instead of having a dad, or two parents, at least I made the best judgment I could in picking someone with good character.

After several insemination attempts with anonymous donor sperm, Sabrina conceived and gave birth to a daughter. When her daughter was about two, she started asking questions about her "donor daddy." At that point, Sabrina's search for more information about her donor intensified, and she started calling the clinic to get more information about him.

SABRINA: So my daughter started asking, "When he smiles does he look like me? Do you think he laughs like me? Do you think I have his eyes?" You know, really detailed questions about would she see herself in this other person. So I asked the clinic to ask him if he could write a more detailed biography, and maybe send a picture or two from when he was younger, or write her a letter without giving away his identity, just to help satisfy her curiosity. Or if he would consider an earlier meeting, if it was driven by my daughter, rather than having to wait until she was eighteen?

It seemed to me my daughter was in pain about having this absence of someone who was such a part of her existence. So initially, according to the clinic, he said he would write something. And I told my daughter it was coming, that he was going to write her a letter, and she was really excited. But he didn't. And she was *really* let down, and that was my bad call.

So, this was over a three-year period and the clinic finally told me his wife was upset and wanted to shut this down because she was frightened about them being found. So the clinic told me, "I think you should consider this a closed book." So I had to let it go and leave it up to my daughter for when she turns eighteen.

But, you know, based on how my daughter feels, when she's at a point where she's more mature and if she comes to me and says, "Mom, I want to meet this guy," I will hire a PI to find him.

I mean, I think it's a sort of disgrace. I'm responsible for my piece of it. I did the best I could with the info I had, but I don't think it's fair to the kids. It's great for the kids who have two parents, of whatever gender, but for the kids who feel like there's a missing element, they have a right to know. And I understand about the donors wanting their privacy and all of that, but I think it's a politically incorrect thing to do, and not very thoughtful of him and his family. And I have my family—my daughter—to deal with. Some kids just need to know who these missing parents are. And for Abby, I see her have this real longing toward men—especially when there are dads around—and I worry about how that long-ing will play out in her life.

But another thing I think about is, say this donor had ten first live births, and then those people are allowed to reserve his sperm so they can have siblings. And I was told that a lot of families come back for seconds. So let's say there are fifteen kids, on the conservative side. Then let's say a lot of them live in San Francisco. That's a lot of goddam siblings. And all in this close proximity. It seems crazy to me that you'd have all these biological half siblings out there and not be able to know who they are. The odds are pretty high they could end up at the same high school, or start dating, and never know they're related. And I've been at some events where I've seen this lesbian couple and they have a daughter who looks exactly like my daughter. And I know they went to the bank. So I wonder if they used the same donor.

So for me, now, it comes down to if someone doesn't feel comfortable about meeting these kids, then maybe they should decide not to be a donor in the first place? I think there needs to be a huge change in the whole reproductive technol-ogy industry—like with adoption now—where it's all out in the open.

DIANE: So how do you think about the donor in terms of what he is and what to call him? Donor? Genetic father?

SABRINA: Having worked with people in the adoption reform movement has really changed how I think. Now, bottom line, he's the father. It's her father. The end.

DIANE: So would you have done anything differently if you could?

SABRINA: Knowing what I know now, I would have waited and used a known donor. Obviously, I wouldn't want any other child than the child I have, but it's hard to see her have so many questions that I can't answer, and to want something I can't give her. I feel responsible for that decision.

Sabrina's experience raises important concerns about using anonymous sperm bank donors as opposed to a known donor that one can trust. For her, the most difficult part is seeing her daughter have questions about her identity that she can-not answer, and she suffered frustrations when she tried to get more information about her donor, to no avail.

THE KIDS ARE ALL RIGHT

There are between thirty thousand and sixty thousand children conceived per year via sperm donation, including children born to single mothers, female-partnered mothers, and heterosexual couples. For most heterosexual couples, deciding when and how to tell a child he or she was donor conceived is difficult because couples are concerned that telling the child will negatively affect the child's relationship with the nonbiological parent (Daniels 2001; Nachtigall et al. 1997). Those who do decide to tell are divided between preferring early disclosure and waiting until

a child has a better understanding of how reproduction works, usually before adolescence (Mac Dougall et al. 2007). For lesbian couples and single women, telling a child he or she was conceived with the help of a sperm donor does not carry
the same emotional weight as it does for straight couples, and single women and
lesbian couples are more inclined to tell their children they were conceived with
donor sperm (Beeson, Jennings, and Kramer 2011; Freeman, Jadva et. al 2009;
Freeman, Zadeh et. al 2016).

Some choose to connect with other families with children conceived from
the same donor, and they perceive others who share the same donor as "linked
families" (Goldberg and Scheib 2015). In the 1990s I attended several holiday
events at The Sperm Bank of California, where families with children conceived
from donors with the sperm bank were able to meet. Connecting children with
their biological half siblings and their respective parents provided an opportunity to experience their shared characteristics and build social connections and
extended kin relations. Contact with same-donor offspring has been shown to be
beneficial to children conceived in this way, especially for enhancing one's sense
of identity (Persaud et al. 2017). For all parents, regardless of sexual orientation
or marital status, the decision to disclose to a child that he or she was donor conceived emerges from the belief that a child has the right to know.

Among eighteen-year-old donor-conceived children who are eligible to get
access to their identity-release donors, those born into single mother or lesbian-
partnered households are more likely to request information about their identity-
release donors than those born to heterosexual couples; women are more
inclined to seek out information or contact with their donors than men; and
94 percent of donor-conceived children plan to contact their donors (Scheib,
Ruby, and Benward 2017). The difference between children born to female-headed
households and those born to heterosexual households could be due to either of
the following reasons: women-headed households are more likely to disclose to
their children how they were conceived than those with a mother and a father
present, or children in heterosexual households who do know they are donor conceived may not feel the need to search out a donor or may not want to compromise the feelings of the father who raised them.

Despite the desire to have more information about one's genetic contributors,
the bulk of the psychosocial literature demonstrates that children born in single
and same-sex-coupled homes grow to be at least as well adjusted and healthy as
those born in more traditional households (Chan, Raboy, and Patterson 1998;
Gartrell and Boss 2010; Biblarz and Stacey 2010). Although there is some evidence
that children with two parents—regardless of whether they are a homosexual or
a heterosexual couple—fare better than children in single-parent households
(Golombok 2015). Most research also demonstrates that disclosure to the child
regarding how he or she was conceived is beneficial to the child (Pasch et al. 2017;
Allan 2016). One study does suggest that adult children conceived via sperm

donation suffer and are disturbed about the nature of their conception (Marquardt, Glenn, and Clark 2010). This study was published by the Institute for American Values and was widely critiqued for its bias against LGBTQ families and lack of scientific rigor.

There is much more data available now on these different family forms than there was in the 1990s. Perceptions surrounding disclosure have changed over time—especially in heterosexual families, which have become more open—but all the reliable data indicate that donor-conceived children suffer no ill effects, regardless of the type of family into which they were born. There appears to be one main caveat, however: donor-conceived children who find out on their own how they were conceived, or are told later—for example, in their teens or twenties—express anger at having been lied to about their biological parentage. When I first started this research in 1990, the children born via sperm donation were still young. Now, however, many have come of age and are able to tell their own stories; they launch or join donor-conceived children social media groups; they use direct-to-consumer genetic test kits; they even launch their own registries to find donors and biologically connected siblings.

Since 2017, I have been able to speak to a number of donor-conceived children, some of whom were conceived from sperm from The Repository for Germinal Choice, others from The Sperm Bank of California, and others from sperm banks or clinics from across the country. These were more informal interviews rather than official research interviews, but I can say that the donor-conceived children who were told from an early age—as is usually the case with same-sex couples and single parents—felt that donor conception was just one part of who they are. The donor-conceived adults who found out later—whether through a genetic test, a nonparent family member, or by one of their parents—expressed significant distress at having been "lied to" about their conception and identities. Some of these people not only felt betrayed, but many also experienced what they referred to as an "identity crisis."

Many donor-conceived people I have spoken to felt compelled to find their donors in order to fill in the missing pieces of their lives. Family structure seems to have little to do with a person's desire to find out more about the donor who helped create them. Some donor-conceived adults do want to form relationships with their donors (and vice versa) and consider them as a type of relative—and some even consider their sperm donors a father. The quest for connection between donors and donor-conceived children poses an interesting anthropological paradox. We often emphasize the social meanings of parenthood—that a parent is someone who chooses to love, raise, and nurture a child. In these conversations, biological definitions of parenthood are diminished in favor of the social role. Yet in most of my conversations with sperm and egg donors—and children conceived with donor sperm or eggs—the significance of biological connection cannot be uniformly erased. Many donor-conceived children, like many children who have been adopted, feel they have a right not only to have information about the person with whom they share half their DNA, but also the opportunity to meet that person if they want to. Donor-connected people find meaning in their genes, to varying degrees.

CONCLUSION

Judith Stacey (1990) addresses how families not defined by traditional gender roles or genetic relatedness have replaced the traditional nuclear family. Family constellations vary—whether formed through adoption, surrogacy, fostering, co-parenting, single parenting, or another process. There are so many different types of families that one could argue the very notion of "alternative family" is obsolete. Regardless of how families are created and structured, the desire to have children is ordinary. Categories of kinship expand—to include donor dads, donor-conceived biological half siblings, and different categories of motherhood—as families are created through technological and legal interventions.

While the term *alternative* may not be useful, there are some significant differences from traditional, nuclear families. Compared to heterosexual, married women, the women in my study without male partners were often met with less than enthusiastic or supportive reactions when they told people about their plans to have a child or revealed that they were pregnant. Day-to-day life for single mothers with unknown donors consisted of the mother being responsible for everything, including income, childcare, and the daily duties of parenting; single mothers with known donors had somewhat more support; for lesbian couples, parenting tasks were shared. Anonymous donors are completely unknown biological contributors with no supportive social roles, but known donors may contribute to the support of their genetic children, but in a very limited way. Known donor support and care for genetic children are usually at the discretion of the mother or mothers—to the degree that their role as "father" may actually be redefined as something else, such as using a more distanced kin term like "uncle" or even "duncle."

Objections to so-called alternative families are embedded in a romanticized notion of the traditional nuclear family consisting of a mother, father, and their children—a standard that has been on a rapid decline since the 1960s. The collapse of the heteronormative family occurred with the simultaneous creation of new family forms, brought about by rising divorce rates, remarriages, live-in heterosexual unmarried households, and the increasing social acceptability of single and lesbian-partnered families. Still, even among single women, the preference for the ideal fantasy family remains, with straight women seeing single motherhood through donor sperm as a last resort in light of their waning reproductive years. Among female-partnered couples, building family via sperm donation replicated, to some degree, heteronormative family structures in the absence of legal marriage, before same-sex marriage was legally recognized. The most radical departures from the heteronormative family structure can be found among women using known donors to create their families. Here, donor dads may have father like relationships with their biological children and supportive relationships with the mothers of those children, but it is the mothers—regardless of sexual orientation or partnership status—who maintain control and authority.

Family, as a universal concept, is defined differently in different cultures. It is not static but rather changes according to place and time and with technological innovations. Sperm and egg provision, embryo donation, mitochondrial DNA replacement, gestational and traditional surrogacy, and as yet unknown possibilities all affect how families are formed and defined, as well as the complicated meanings underlying social, spatial, and genetic parenthood. While traditional family is in many ways a romanticized idea of the past, for many the ideals of lifelong partnership and procreation within that partnership remain strong, regardless of sexual orientation. Anthropological studies on the impact of assisted reproductive technologies and family can lead to new insights into how family and kinship are defined, the significance of different kinds of parenthood (genetic, social, gestational, and spatial), and how the rise of new family forms contributes to broader changes to social, medical, and legal institutions—including marriage.

9 · FROM MURPHY BROWN
TO MODERN FAMILIES

John Arthur was dying. Struck by ALS, with little time left, he had a last wish: that his husband and partner of twenty years, Jim Obergefell, would be able to have his name entered on his death certificate as his surviving spouse. He wanted Jim to be legally taken care of after his passing, as any spouse would (Cenziper and Obergefell 2016). The couple had married on a plane in Maryland in 2013, outfitted with the medical equipment necessary to keep John comfortable. Several months after their wedding, John passed away. But the battle to honor his dying wish endured.

In 2015, after years of legal wrangling through the court system, in the case *Obergefell v. Hodges*, the U.S. Supreme Court ruled in favor of Obergefell.[1] Same-sex couples could now marry and—in theory—enjoy all the same rights offered to married couples. But could they?

Same-sex married couples now have some of the rights heterosexual married couples have—health insurance benefits, spouse's name on state records, joint tax returns—but when it comes to the "presumption of parentage," the *Obergefell* decision is silent.

Amid the celebrations of this landmark Supreme Court decision, I thought about the women in same-sex partnerships I interviewed back in the 1990s. I recalled Bonnie and Sharon's story about caseworkers who came to their home and assessed their suitability as a family so that an Alameda County judge, with his gavel of approval, would legally recognize both of them as parents. I also thought about all the women who lost custody of their children either because they left a heterosexual partnership for a lesbian relationship or because they had children in a lesbian relationship that ended and they were the nonbiological mother.

When I first heard about the *Obergefell* decision, I assumed it would eliminate the need for second-parent adoption and automatically protect the rights of both parents in same-sex marriages, regardless of biological connection. Instead, the presumption of parentage is still open to interpretation at the state level.

Forty-eight states recognize the presumption of parenthood clause, but Arkansas and Indiana do not, leaving homosexual parents and the children born into those unions in those states in legal limbo. Several states and the District of Columbia grant parental recognition even if the parents are not in a legally recognized union. The *Obergefell* decision has had a ripple effect on a range of other cases related to LGBTQ family building.

Despite its shortcomings, the *Obergefell* decision represents an enormous shift in thinking about marriage and family from the 1990s to today. This shift has been accompanied by changes in popular culture, social attitudes, language, policy, access to medical care, and advanced technologies that influence how families are created and identified. For example, the popular television sitcom *Murphy Brown* pushed the boundaries regarding the social acceptance of single motherhood in the 1990s and sparked a conservative "family values" backlash. Interestingly, in light of the rising Trump conservativism, the hit series is making a comeback. A more recent television sitcom, *Modern Family*, demonstrates the changing configurations of family—including a married, gay couple and their Vietnamese adopted daughter. Interestingly, even though the Republican platform largely opposes same-sex marriage, *Modern Family* has not spawned the same kind of conservative response that *Murphy Brown* did over two decades ago. In fact, Ann Romney, the wife of former Republican presidential candidate Mitt Romney, said it was her "favorite show" (Serwer 2012). Other shows, like *The Fosters* and *The L Word*, also depict a range of family constellations.

"Modern families"—single-parent families, same-sex two-parent families, families that have been recombined through divorce and remarriage (or unmarried partners), and families created via donor egg, donor sperm, or surrogacy (Golombok 2015)—have gained wider social acceptance. In 2006, the Ethics Committee of the American Society for Reproductive Medicine (ASRM) recommended that gays, lesbians, and unmarried persons not be denied access to fertility treatment, stating, "There is no persuasive evidence that children raised by single parents or by gays and lesbians are harmed or disadvantaged," and all requests for assisted reproduction should be treated equally (2006, 1334). The committee issued a similar statement in 2013 (Ethics Committee of the ASRM 2013), which marked a significant shift in the treatment of single and LGBTQ families and encouraged fertility specialists to treat all patients equally, regardless of marital status, sexual orientation, or gender identification (Ethics Committee of the ASRM 2015).

In order to address some of the more recent changes since I first started down this research path over two decades ago, I conducted some new interviews and some follow-up interviews and included some observations from my recent research on egg donors and the egg donation industry. For anthropologists doing research at home, it is often difficult to decide when to stop, but the advantage is that you can easily check back in with the community you worked with.

MARRIAGE EQUALITY AND MODERN FAMILIES

In 2000, California Proposition 22, which passed by a wide margin, defined marriage as between a man and a woman only. In February 2004, San Francisco mayor Gavin Newsom asked the county clerk to issue marriage licenses to same-sex couples who applied for them. Immediately, same-sex couples rushed to city hall to have their relationships legally recognized. The Campaign for California Families and the Proposition 22 Legal Defense Fund immediately filed suit to prevent the city from issuing licenses to same-sex couples, and ultimately San Francisco sued the State of California to stop issuing marriage licenses to same-sex couples. By August, the California Supreme Court had voided San Francisco same-sex marriages. In September 2005, the California Senate passed a bill recognizing same-sex marriage, which Governor Arnold Schwarzenegger promptly vetoed. On May 15, 2008, the California Supreme Court lifted the ban, and between June 16 and November 8, 2008, over eighteen thousand same-sex couples were married. In November 2008, Proposition 8 passed, which defined marriage as between a man and a woman.[2] Two years later, Proposition 8 was struck down, but in the meantime, the eighteen thousand couples were left in legal limbo until the *Obergefell* decision.

By June 2009, Governor Schwarzenegger and Attorney General Jerry Brown declined to defend the constitutionality of Proposition 8. "Taking from same-sex couples the right to civil marriage that they had previously possessed under California's Constitution cannot be squared with guarantees of the Fourteenth Amendment," Attorney General Brown stated. By 2011, federal judge James Walker had struck down Proposition 8 as unconstitutional. The Supreme Court then struck down the Defense of Marriage Act and dismissed Proposition 8 in June 2012, and lifted the ban on gay marriage. The legal wrangling continued in California, largely being decided in favor of same-sex couples, until the *Obergefell* decision put the issue to rest at the federal level in 2015. Although this was an enormous win for marriage equality, many in the community continue to feel their relationships, families, and futures remain in jeopardy and that their rights are fragile— including the right to reproduce.

Maya, fifty-one, was raised in a commune in the 1970s. Her mother was a single parent who divorced her dad when Maya was three. Talking about her childhood, Maya told me, "I was raised in a community of adults, who loved me, whether or not they were genetically related. And they were good to me. In that commune I actually had love and care and attention in a way that was more functional than a nuclear family." Her experiences growing up have had a profound impact on her and how she sees family and community now.

I met Maya at a Berkeley café in June 2017. We had first met several years earlier, when I worked at a nonprofit organization in Berkeley and she was hosting an event on LGBTQ family-building options. She has been active in the LGBTQ community in the Bay Area, has worked for many years to educate people in her community about assisted reproductive technology options, and has been involved in grassroots organizing to change policies surrounding LGBTQ family-building. She and her partner, Chino—who is transmasculine and butch identified—have been together for twenty years.[3] Maya gave birth to their daughter in 2004, with sperm from a known, multiethnic, gay donor with ancestry that matches Chino's Chinese Mexican ancestry. Maya, who has Scotch Irish ancestry, and Chino represent a truly intersectional family that unites varied gender and ethnic identities.

Maya and Chino have lived through the biopolitical swings in the state of California. The debates over marriage and family equality are not abstract moral arguments for Maya; they are a fight for rights that heterosexual people take for granted, and that directly impact her body, her family, her community, and her life. I asked Maya how the *Obergefell* decision and the marriage equality movement more broadly affected her family and the people she knows. She responded,

> I don't know necessarily if there was a big "gayby" boom after, but there certainly was a marriage boom. Marriage rights and parental protections are significant—people who are now married are accessing health care and having that coverage really helps with people who want to have children.
>
> For us, the marriage equality movement was a big part of the story in my daughter's conception story because I was two months pregnant when we got married the first time in city hall, in 2004. My partner called me and said, "Hey do you wanna get married? Turn on the news, they're actually legally marrying LGBTQ folks at city hall."
>
> And in a way we were participating in civil disobedience. It was a big deal and very profound and being pregnant and forming a family. And in August of that year when our marriages were annulled along with 4,038 other families it was very, very humiliating, angering.
>
> For me, marriage wasn't even really on the top of my list as an activist, partly because I didn't believe in the institution of marriage. I thought it was a regressive institution and I was a feminist. So having that experience made me want to bring the voices of families like ours, voices of LGBTQ and people of color communities, voices of working-class communities. Before that the voices around the marriage equality movement were primarily white, middle class, mostly childless, cis gay male.
>
> And right now, I'm afraid, we're in a terrible time under the current [Trump] administration. I read the other day about a lesbian married couple in Indiana. People who conceived with sperm from sperm banks are losing their rights as parents and sperm donors fighting for custody are winning. The more marginalized parents are, the more we are worried about our rights being chipped away at.

Maya has personally experienced the changing political and legal definitions of her relationship. Marriage became a political act. Her experience demonstrates that hard-won rights cannot be taken for granted, as they can easily be taken away if or when the wind changes.

The state has power over both marriage and family. In addition to the lengthy battle over marriage equality, same-sex couples face ongoing challenges that undermine the security of their families. As Jennifer Reich (2005) demonstrates, those who live outside conventional norms are vulnerable to state interventions that can deny them the right to parent their own children. These legal battles take many forms. In a recent case in Kansas, after genetic tests confirmed biological paternity, the state sued William Marotta, a man who provided sperm for a lesbian couple, to provide child support for the child conceived from his sperm. The court stated that Marotta—a sperm donor who answered a Craigslist ad posted by a lesbian couple—was a "presumptive parent" because his sperm did not pass through a licensed physician before it was used for home insemination. When the couple split and one of the partners filed for social services, the state wanted Marotta to pay child support instead. He appealed and eventually won his case in November 2016.[4]

In New Jersey, Sheena and Tiara Yates, an African American lesbian couple, conceived two sons from two different known sperm donors using home insemination. Each donor separately sued the Yateses for partial custody and visitation, despite having both signed contracts in which they relinquished parental rights. In both cases, the court decided against the Yateses and determined that the donors were entitled to visitation rights. Other donors have been winning visitation rights as well (Culhane 2015). These sorts of cases continue to be brought even after the U.S. Supreme Court has recognized the rights of all couples to marry because there still is no uniform legal protection should they decide to procreate within that marriage. There is some evidence that this is beginning to change, however.

Some states, including California, Iowa, Kansas, and Utah, now permit same-sex parents to both be named as parents on their children's birth certificates. California now has liberal protections for LGBTQ families, compared to many other states. As of January 1, 2016, California birth certificates included the gender-neutral term *parent* on birth certificates, rather than the exclusive terms *mother* and *father*. In many states, such as Wisconsin and North Carolina, lawsuits are pending for this right. In one such case in Indiana, a married lesbian couple sought to have both mothers' names on their daughter's birth certificate. The State of Indiana appealed to overturn a district judge's decision ordering the state to recognize both women as parents on the birth certificate. In May 2017, Judge Diane Sykes, who presided over the case, determined that "you can't overcome biology" and that since the "paternity presumption is impossible in same-sex marriage," there is no discrimination (Wang 2017). In their case, the couple argued that parental recognition should be covered under the *Obergefell* ruling.

On June 26, 2017, in a similar case before the U.S. Supreme Court, *Pavan v. Smith*, the court stated that, as explained in *Obergefell*, "The Constitution entitles same-sex couples to civil marriage on the same terms and conditions as opposite-sex couples." It further stated that among the "rights, benefits, and responsibilities to which same-sex couples, no less than opposite-sex couples, must have access— we expressly identified 'birth and death certificates.'"[5] This decision makes it clear that states cannot discriminate against same-sex couples, whether it is in recognizing their marriages or upholding their rights to have their families recognized.

While the *Obergefell* decision does offer some protections in same-sex family recognition, the rights of nonbiological parents are still vulnerable—especially given that different courts and different states interpret decisions differently. In June 2017, in *Turner v. Oakley*, Turner filed for divorce and sought full custody of the child she and Oakley conceived and delivered during their marriage. Turner is the biological mother. The Arizona Court of Appeals ruled that Oakley, a nonbiological mother, was not a legal parent—even though she and her partner were married, they planned and conceived a child within their relationship, and both partners' names were on their child's birth certificate—because she had not legally adopted the child. In its decision, the court argued that the *Obergefell* decision was irrelevant because it had nothing to do with parenting statutes, and that the "presumption of parenthood" had to do with paternity and does not mandate gender neutrality.[6] At the time of this writing, Oakley is appealing the case. Many of these cases still come down to gendered, binary language, which assumes paternity regardless of biological connection to offspring in heterosexual couples but prioritizes biological parenthood over social parenthood in same-sex couples with children.

Same-sex couples and their children face substantial challenges in having their families recognized and protected by the law. While there are some positive trends in terms of marriage equality, presumption of parenthood and child custody issues remain unsettled. Still, even with hard-fought gains in marriage and parenting rights, same-sex couples and their children live under ongoing threat that laws may change under different administrations. Without the same legal recognition that heterosexual couples have, same-sex partners and their children are left vulnerable—especially given how laws vary from state to state. For same-sex partners with children, going through the second-parent adoption process is essential in order to protect the relationship between a nonbiological parent and his or her child, regardless of whether one's state allows for both partners' names to be listed on a birth certificate. From state to state, definitions of parenthood vary, causing some parents not to be fully recognized as the parents of their children, depending on the state in which they live.

ASSISTED REPRODUCTIVE TECHNOLOGIES, MARRIAGE EQUALITY, AND THE SPERM-BANKING INDUSTRY

I reconnected with Barbara Raboy at the underground Berkeley Jazz School Café, adjacent to the Berkeley Jazz School, on a cool Thursday evening in 2017. We were both a bit older but recognized each other immediately. She had rehearsal that night for a jazz ensemble, where she plays the saxophone. Barbara stepped down as executive director of the Sperm Bank of California (TSBC) in 2000 to pursue other opportunities, but she remained on their board until 2005. Before we met, I sent her a copy of some of the chapters I had written that included my interviews with her because I wanted to make sure I represented her words accurately. I also wanted to ask her some follow-up questions. She suggested I also talk to Alice Ruby, who became executive director of TSBC in 2002. Barbara now enjoys her retirement.

I returned to the Berkeley office building TSBC has called home since 1995. As I pressed the elevator button to go up to the second floor, I thought of Rebecca—and many other women—who shared with me the physical and emotional sensations she experienced when she went in for "sperm pick up." On the ride up in the elevator, I thought about all the people—prospective parents and sperm donors—who had pushed that same button and ridden in that same elevator, and whose sperm, eggs, and uteruses had combined to make children, whether they are aware of each other or not. I wondered, How many children have resulted from these different trips up the elevator? After I exited the elevator, the receptionist led me to a conference room—the same conference room I had sat in years ago while attending TSBC-sponsored seminars on conceiving through donor insemination and the legal paths for same-sex families to have their parental rights recognized. As I sat and waited for Alice, I noticed that a statistic had been written on the whiteboard in red marker: over four thousand children have been born as a result of TSBC.

Alice entered the conference room and sat down at the table, coffee cup in hand. With a master's in public health, she has been working on women's health issues since college. Like many others I have spoken to throughout the years who work in this industry, her work is also personal: "I'm a lesbian mom and have a known donor for my son. I started out as a single mom. I'm also the adult child of a queer parent. My mom came out when I was in elementary school and left my dad and has been with women since then, and my brother was adopted. So I've had a long-term connection to nontraditional family that I think is really beneficial in my work. So the organization is a good fit for me. It feels like a calling."

I asked Alice what kinds of changes she had seen since 2002—almost two years after my last visit there, when I left some flyers to recruit sperm donors for my research. She responded,

I've seen a lot of changes in the industry. One has to do with the technological changes. After ICSI [intracytoplasmic sperm injection] came along, a lot of men who would have used sperm donors with their wives were now using ICSI and their own sperm—it was more expensive, but they did.

This meant all those sperm banks and practices that weren't so comfortable with single moms or two-mom families suddenly became more comfortable. Someone who works at another sperm bank came up to me at a conference and said, "You know, we're going after your market now." And I read a quote from someone else who works at a large sperm bank that said, "A lot of people around here got real progressive, real fast." Suddenly the sperm banks—all of them—had to reckon with the fact that they couldn't just serve this one population.

ICSI is a technology that allows an embryologist to select a single sperm and, under magnification, inject it into an egg to fertilize it. The first child born from ICSI was in Belgium in 1992 (Van Steirteghem 2012), and like all emerging reproductive technologies, it took a number of years before it gained widespread use. This technology enabled people with a low sperm count, low motility, or abnormally shaped sperm to fertilize an egg. Even men who had vasectomies could still father a child, as even a single sperm cell could be surgically removed from the testicles to inject into an egg. For heterosexual couples, this was an enormous advance in technology that enabled men with male-factor infertility to have a biological child with their partner, rather than using a sperm donor.

As Alice mentioned, this one technological innovation changed the entire sperm-banking industry. All the sperm banks that served heterosexual couples exclusively—or even primarily—could no longer operate unless they changed their business plan. For many of these sperm banks, the decision to provide services to single women and lesbian couples was not due to an ideological shift but rather was made out of financial necessity in order to keep their doors open for business. TSBC only saw their business from heterosexual couples drop from about 18 percent of their clientele to around 14 percent. Single women increased from about 20 percent of their clients to around 40 percent, and lesbian and queer couples remained around 60 percent of their clientele.

According to Alice, same-sex marriage has also had an impact on the business and altered the profile of people who come to TSBC for donor sperm:

Historically, the majority of our moms were over the age of thirty-five. But more recently, we're seeing in the last ten years or so, as same-sex marriage is becoming more accepted nationally, and more people are getting married and getting married younger, we're seeing more lesbian couples in their early thirties or late twenties, whereas before it was very rare to see someone come in here in their twenties.

At the same time, we're still seeing a lot of single moms come in here trending older. For the older single moms, it's plan B or C for them, regardless of their sexual orientation. But most of the single moms are heterosexual—85 to 90 percent.

For women in their late thirties, early forties, a lot of them are using their own eggs. In midforties or later, they're using donor eggs, or possibly eggs that they've frozen or embryos they've created.

Interestingly, same-sex marriage rights appear to influence the age at which couples decide to start their families, with lesbian couples coming in for donor sperm earlier than single women. This is at a time when the average age of heterosexual first-time mothers is going up (Matthews and Hamilton 2016). Single women, regardless of sexual orientation, are still coming in during their mid- to late thirties, as most still hold out hope that they will have a child with a partner. Some older sperm bank clients take advantage of relatively newer—and more expensive—technologies and use donor sperm with their own frozen and thawed eggs, with a donor egg, or with embryos created from donor sperm. These options were not as easily available in the 1990s. Despite ongoing challenges to legal protections for same-sex couples and their children, marriage equality has had a significant positive impact on the LGBTQ community.

The meaning of marriage has changed significantly over time, shifting from a focus on economic security, institutions, producing children, and binding groups together before the Industrial Revolution to an increased focus on love and companionship at the beginning of the twentieth century (Burgess and Locke 1945; Kimport 2014). According to Stephanie Coontz (2005), marriage has become more individualistic, and it does not organize people's lives in the same way it has historically (Cherlin 2004). Contemporary meanings for different-sex couples and same-sex couples are parallel—to affirm "commitment, interdependency and love" (Kimport 2014, 73).

Marriage rights for same-sex couples reflect changing social attitudes toward relationship diversity, even in a rocky political environment. The *Obergefell* decision was every bit as significant for same-sex couples as was the U.S. Supreme Court *Loving v. Virginia* decision for civil rights and interracial marriage.[7] However, in the *Loving* decision, as married heterosexual partners, couples had the right to procreate and have their children recognized as their own. For same-sex couples, even if they are married, parenting rights are not assumed because people are of necessity creating children via third-party reproduction, where someone outside the relationship has a biological connection to the child. The next step beyond *Obergefell* will undoubtedly speak to legal recognition of, and protection for, same-sex parents and their offspring at a federal level.

FRESH SPERM, THE FOOD AND DRUG ADMINISTRATION, AND REGULATING SEX

Through Maya, I reconnected with Leland, founder of Rainbow Flag Health Services (RFHS). He retired in 2012 and I no longer had his contact information, but I wanted to follow up and ask him why he closed RFHS and what changes he had observed since we first spoke, over two decades prior. Maya first met Leland in 2009, when she and her partner, Chino, sought fertility treatment with their known donor for a second child. Maya and Chino's numerous attempts to conceive via home inseminations proved unsuccessful, and Maya wanted to pursue the next step in assisted reproduction using intrauterine insemination (IUI) with her known donor's sperm. For IUI, the sperm has to be washed before insemination to remove prostaglandins from the semen that may cause an adverse reaction in the uterus. Basically, the process separates the sperm from the semen that contains it.

She had a difficult time finding a doctor who would do the insemination because Food and Drug Administration (FDA) regulations prohibited IUI with fresh sperm from "nonintimate partners." The FDA only permitted the use of frozen sperm that had been quarantined for six months. Maya finally found an LGBTQ-friendly physician who would perform the procedure for her, but she needed to have the sperm washed elsewhere before she could be inseminated with it. She, her partner, and their donor would meet at RFHS, where Leland would wash the sperm, and then she would take it to her doctor—over an hour away in traffic—to do the insemination.

I met Leland at his home, above a shop on a tree-lined street in Alameda. He and I talked for a while, and Maya joined us later. I asked Leland about the trends he saw in the industry.

> One of the things I noticed was fewer and fewer people wanted to buy sperm and more and more were asking a friend to be a sperm donor. And an increasing number of my clients were people who came to me with a sperm donor, and the vast majority of them were doing inseminations at home, despite the fact that there was no legal protection at that time for home insemination. They trusted the donors to relinquish parental rights so their partner could adopt.
>
> The problem was that, although they had been doing home insemination, the FDA has regulations that said that unless you were sexually intimate partners, you couldn't do fresh insemination. They certainly were free to do what they wanted at home, but that constrained licensed medical professionals from doing fresh IUI.
>
> The FDA tried to make it illegal for gay men to be sperm donors. They did two things. One, they came out with a guidance document that said, "Don't use gay men as sperm donors." Now at the top of every page it said, "This is not regulation, this is suggestion only." Nonetheless, people who owned sperm banks inter-

preted those guidance documents as if they were regulations. Some people would swear to me up and down this was part of the regulation, but it wasn't.

The FDA intimidated people. Since they knew they couldn't get a ban on gay sperm donors into regulations, legally they knew it would be challenged, but they put it into this guidance document knowing that if it went in front of a court the judge would say, "Well this isn't enforceable law." But de facto it was. It intimidated everyone—except me and a few others—into not accepting gay sperm donors.

So I was inspected by the FDA. And every time I asked the inspector, "Can you enforce a guidance document as if it is regulation?" And they would say, "No, no, no, you can't do that." Then two weeks later they would call me up and say, "You're using gay men as donors." And I would say, "Yes, it's perfectly legal." Then they would send me threatening letters saying, "You're in violation." And I would ask, "What violation?" And they sent me to the website and it was just go to the guidance document. So it was intimidation.

They were trying to get their way with anonymous donations the way they tried to get their way with fresh donations. They said unless you were sexually intimate partners you had to get tested seven days prior to the insemination. Lab tests usually take four to five days to process. And a woman doesn't always know exactly when she's ovulating, and sometimes it might come a little later. So if she ovulates early, on Monday, and he doesn't have his lab results back yet, you can't do the insemination. If she ovulates late, and goes beyond the seven days, you can't do the insemination. So they thought they had me on this one.

So it made me think. One of the terms they did not define was "sexually intimate partner" because they thought it was self-evident. So I said, if people were inseminating at home, they were already exposed to the man's bodily fluids, and therefore from a public health point of view—not a legal or social point of view—they already were sexually intimate partners.

I was getting to the point where I wanted to retire. I was just getting tired. The FDA harassment, the emotional intensity of what I was doing, working alone, it was exhausting. But I couldn't retire because I was literally the only person in California aboveboard who was doing fresh IUI with directed donors. So, I figured, what would convince somebody? Changing the law.

Leland set out to change the California law that defined the meaning of *sexually intimate partner* when it came to fertility treatment. He connected with the National Center for Lesbian Rights and Equality California as sponsoring organizations, and together they contacted Maya to testify and organize around the bill. Then–assembly member Nancy Skinner agreed to author the bill, AB 2356, that sought to clarify the definition of *sexually intimate partner* to recognize people using fresh sperm with known donors. Kaiser and the California Medical Association also signed on in support of the bill. It passed through the assembly and the senate, and Governor Jerry Brown signed it into law in September 2012.

After winning this broader definition of *sexually intimate partner*, people were able to get treatment using fresh sperm from known donors at Kaiser and other fertility care providers in the state of California. This expanded definition in California ended up having an impact on the FDA. Leland continued,

> My argument was if a man and woman are going into a house to inseminate, it is none of the FDA's business whether they have sex, or whether he ejaculates into a cup and she goes into another room and inseminates herself. The end result is the same. And if the FDA is going to say one thing is not covered and the other was, then the FDA becomes the sex police. And that is not their role.
>
> So California had this new policy defining "sexually intimate partners" [SIP]. And not too long after that I saw letters the FDA sent to people where they essentially acknowledge our definition of SIP, and I don't know if the FDA knows it came from me, but now they can no longer discriminate between people who are having sex and people who are using fresh donor sperm to get pregnant.

Maya arrived at Leland's house as he and I talked about changes in California laws that were more hospitable to LGBTQ families. She spoke to Leland about her appreciation for his work and what the passage of AB 2356 meant to her.

MAYA: As someone who went through eight years of trying to have another child, and the very devastating experience of getting access to IUI as a lesbian and working-class person with health insurance who paid out of pocket, you [Leland] were the only provider in Northern California who would serve us with fresh unquarantined sperm. I knew it was discriminatory, you knew it was discriminatory, and everyone we had gone to for treatment but who wouldn't do the inseminations knew it was discriminatory. It was just so wrong that we were paying out of pocket. We were going into debt. We were driving over to San Ramon to get the ultrasound and HCG shots because those were covered by insurance. We were driving to Alameda to have our donor meet us at Leland's office to get the donor's sperm and IUIs, and then going back to San Ramon to get testing.

And I knew, as an organizer, I knew passing AB 2356 wasn't going to help us. My eggs were done. So I could speak from the grief and the struggle and the frustrations of that process and I knew it wasn't going to change my family-building story, but I recognized we were your patients and then we were comrades in the legislature. And I knew this would help other people behind me on their conception journeys.

LELAND: When I went to Reno I ran into a friend of one of my godsons. And he's now doing a fresh insemination as a directed donor at Kaiser. At Kaiser! I said you're doing that because of our work. They'll never know our names, and maybe that's how it should be, but now thousands of people are doing this because of our work.

After his legislative victory, Leland closed the doors to Rainbow Flag, knowing this single piece of legislation would change the lives of people who wanted to use known donors, as well as reduce the need for the services RFHS provided. In his retirement, he spends time with his kids and husband, takes acting and ballet classes, and, at sixty-five, is attending law school.

FROM DONOR DADS TO GAY DADS

Many of the gay known sperm donors I talked to saw sperm donation as their only path to quasi-parenthood. Less than a father and more than a donor, many of these men referred to themselves or were referred to as donor dads, uncles, or fathers, depending on the degree of relationship they had with the children and their mothers. It was mostly the mothers—who were the legal parents and guardians— who defined these relationships, especially when their children were young. For many gay men in the 1990s, this was one of the few ways they could have a biological child and have some involvement in that child's life, even though they would not be the parent. Stigma in the United States and abroad against gay men and same-sex male couples meant adoption was rarely an option, and international adoption was a costly alternative.

Shortly after I last saw Leland in 1999, he and his partner adopted a son. In 2005, they had a daughter through traditional surrogacy—they used Leland's sperm to inseminate the surrogate directly, using her own eggs. They spent $41,000 on the process. While most people spend upwards of six figures for surrogacy, Leland and his husband were able to get a reduced cost because of his work and connections in the fertility business. Leland talked about his personal experience of becoming a dad and changes he has seen in the industry over the years.

> Our son, who is adopted, is seventeen now, and just graduated high school. Adoption can also be very expensive. In California now, adoption is just as available to gay men as it is to everyone else, but back then it was pretty difficult if you weren't heterosexual and married.
>
> So we had our second child through surrogacy. And last year we went and visited our daughter's surrogate and spent some time with her and her two sons. And then we drove down the coast further and visited a gay couple who also used her as a surrogate with her eggs. So we visited her two sons and then this other couple and their son who are the biological half siblings of our daughter. If my daughter wants to have contact with her she can.

For Leland and his family, it was important for their daughter to have that connection to her surrogate and biological half siblings.

In addition to more options for family creation—for gay men, lesbian couples, and transgender people—having their relationships legally recognized has had a significant impact on their lives and family stability. Leland continued,

> One of the things I have noticed is the vast majority of lesbian couples I know, the nonbiological mother feels very nervous—particularly if there's a known donor. They're like, "Who am I? I'm not related to the kid."
>
> I think now that the legal situation is cleared up in California—and this was before federal recognition of same-sex marriage—now the nonbiological mothers are legally protected, it gives them more solace and support. So I think it has offered us more stability.
>
> There's also a psychological component. Stewart and I have been together twenty-seven years. And we've been legally married for three and a half years. He started calling me his husband a quarter century ago. But he says now that we're legally married it feels different for him.
>
> We waited until October 11, 2015, to get married, which was National Coming Out Day, and it was the twenty-second anniversary of when we first signed domestic partnerships in the city of Berkeley. So we got legally married on our twenty-second anniversary. And our daughter was eight years old at the time and our kids were at the ceremony and my daughter said to me, "You mean you had children before you got married?"

Same-sex marriage rights on the national level, coupled with California laws recognizing parental rights for both partners in a same-sex couple, have improved the overall security of same-sex-parent families. Nonbiological mothers in California now have a more legally secure relationship with the children born into their relationships than they did a couple of decades ago—but this protection is not nationwide, leaving many nonbiological lesbian mothers in legal limbo. For couples like Leland and his husband, legal recognition of their family also offers more comfort for their children.

Some LGBTQ people prefer to adopt or foster a child, and they turn to fertility treatment after hitting logistical, legal, and social barriers preventing them from adopting. For most people, regardless of marital status and sexual orientation, adoption is not usually a first choice. As Leland states, "I think most human beings, whether heterosexual or queer, have a tendency to want a biological child." This desire for a biological child has always dominated heterosexual couples' decisions on their path through fertility treatment before choosing adoption as a way to parenthood. But, as Merit Melhuus (2012) discusses, how people think about one's "own child" may shift according to the substances (eggs, sperm), processes (interior or exterior conception and gestation), and practices (adopting, feeding, raising) used in creating that child.

Until recently, many gay men did not even see parenthood as an option. According to Leland, one of the most significant changes he has seen in the gay community is that gay men now think about children and family in a way they did not before.

I think what's happened is more of a social shift that more and more gay men are being asked to be known donors and more and more are saying yes. I ask young gay men, do you think you'll ever have kids, and they say, "Yeah I think I'll have kids." But men my generation, they didn't think about it at all. I remember some older gay men came to our house and when I talked to them about wanting to have a kid, they thought I was nuts. Of course, it was forty-seven years ago. And they were like, "Oh are you going to get married and pretend you're straight? You're gonna have to get married if you want to have kids." And I was like, "No I'm not going to get married. I'm not going to pretend I'm straight. But I still plan to have kids." They thought I was a Martian. That's totally changed.

In her book *Gay Fatherhood*, Ellen Lewin (2009) challenges the stereotype that gay men prefer pleasure over responsibility and do not actively pursue fatherhood. In the 1990s, for gay men, becoming a known donor was one of the easiest paths to becoming at least a partial father, but that option did not give them full parental autonomy. Coming back to the sitcom *Modern Family*, characters Cam and Mitchell adopt their baby girl from Vietnam. For years, adoption was one of the main ways same-sex male couples created their families; single people and heterosexual couples also sought out children from abroad. In the 1990s, there was an adoption explosion, especially for Chinese and Russian children, but by 2004, international adoptions declined by nearly 50 percent. Many international adoption agencies stopped permitting same-sex couples to adopt children altogether. Since 2007, China has prohibited single people, homosexual people, and trans people from adopting Chinese children.

As Lewin points out, with new assisted reproductive technology options, such as egg donation and surrogacy, many same-sex male couples are able to pursue having children in a way that was not available to them before. International adoption and third-party procreative technology allowed gay men to create families where they were in control as the primary parents. In my most recent research with egg donors, many stated that they provided eggs specifically with the intent of helping gay couples have their own children. Technological innovations are having a profound effect on the way LGBTQ families are formed. At the same time, while advances in assisted reproductive technologies enhance options for family creation, they also raise concerns about the health impact on women who provide eggs and wombs. Additionally, the domestic and international market for egg providers and gestational surrogates evokes a range of ethical dilemmas, including:

the imbalance of class and power between those who provide reproductive services and those who can pay for these services, the meanings of informed consent when decisions to provide eggs or gestate another person's child are driven by poverty, and the rights of children born via third party arrangements.

ASSISTED REPRODUCTIVE TECHNOLOGIES BEYOND BINARY IDENTITIES

In addition to the changes in family structure, there has been a marked shift in how we think about gender and sex and the language we use to define how people identify. In "Traffick in Women," anthropologist Gayle Rubin (1996) addresses how the sex/gender system imposes a false division on society, and she calls for an androgynous and genderless society devoid of false gender hierarchies. Instead of perpetuating male-female binaries, our language has shifted to address the spectrum of difference in people's lived experience. A person whose identity and gender correspond with the individual's sex at birth is now referred to as "cis"; a cis male is someone who identifies as a man and has male genitalia, while a cis female is someone who identifies as a woman and has female genitalia. Being cis identified does not necessarily mean one is heterosexual. One can identify as a cis lesbian woman, for example. A person who has male genitalia and sperm may not identify as a man and could be a trans woman. An individual with ovaries and a uterus may not identify as a woman and could be a trans man. Some people identify as nonbinary. Some trans people undergo surgeries to change their bodies to match their identities; some do not. Some people take hormones so their bodies better match their identities; some do not. How people experience their sexuality and gender in relation to the body they were born in is complicated, and our language is evolving to address these nuances. Increased awareness of trans identities and concerns has also entered into the assisted reproductive technology arena.

When I started this research, I focused on single women and lesbian couples having children through donor insemination. I was aware there is a spectrum of sexual identities and orientations—including heterosexual, bisexual, lesbian, and queer, and a range of terms, including *dyke, butch, femme,* and *trans.* While the category of women without male partners pursuing motherhood through donor insemination seemed straightforward, I discovered the reality is much more complex.

Even the idea of a "sperm donor" turned out to be much more complicated than I initially thought. Some were sperm bank donors, some were known donors, and some known donors were technically and legally fathers because they had sexual relations with the intended mother. In the 1990s, I pushed normative boundaries by exploring technology-assisted reproduction outside the confines of heterosexual, married relationships. At the time, there was very little research on single women and same-sex female couples having kids, but there was also virtually no awareness about transgender people and their reproductive needs.

The past five years have seen a significant rise in transgender awareness, with Bruce Jenner's decision to become Caitlyn Jenner being one of the most high-profile cases. Laverne Cox became the first openly transgender actor to receive a Prime Time Emmy Award for her portrayal of trans woman prisoner Sophia Burset, on Netflix's American comedy-drama *Orange Is the New Black*. Thomas Beatie, a transgender man, became pregnant by donor insemination in 2007, due to his wife's infertility.[8] In September 2016, Evan Hempel, a transgender man who was born female and chose not to undergo sexual correction surgery, also conceived and gave birth to a son using donor sperm.[9] Studies show that transgender parents and their children have positive relationships and children of transgender parents have positive outcomes (Stotzer, Herman, and Hasenbush 2014).

In some countries, in order to change one's name on a birth certificate, driver's license, or other document, sterilization is compulsory. Indeed, in France and twenty-two other European countries, transgender people were not permitted by law to change their names on their driver's licenses and birth certificates unless they had undergone sterilization surgery. On April 6, 2017, the European Court of Human Rights agreed with gay and transgender activists that forced sterilization of transgender people constitutes a human rights violation and issued a ruling in their favor.[10]

Transgender and intersex people have existed throughout time and across cultures. But in many societies, largely due to stigma and discrimination, transgender issues have only recently come to light, and trans reproductive concerns are part of that conversation. Forced sterilization of transgender people is another important reproductive justice and human rights issue, with eugenic implications.

Transgender identities complicate how we think about gender, sexuality, and reproduction. For example, a transgender person can now medically manage his or her body in order to live in a body that resembles the gender with which the individual identifies but also still be able to experience the reproductive capacity of the body the person was born into. Through medical treatment and reproductive technologies, fathers can give birth and mothers can provide sperm. While people with a range of identities have always existed and are present across cultures, increased awareness has fundamentally challenged how we think about categories of parenthood, biology, and identity.

Alice (from TSBC) explained how the shift toward increased trans awareness has affected the sperm bank business:

ALICE: We've been storing sperm for individuals who identify as trans for a very long time. They would come to the sperm bank and freeze their sperm before starting their hormones to transition, so they could use it to get a partner pregnant in the future.

But what's been happening over the past five years is seeing more recipients who are trans. At first we were seeing more partners, who were usually female to male, and their partners were being inseminated with donor sperm. But now we're starting to see female-to-male recipients who are themselves trying to conceive with donor sperm. So they identify as male but they want to conceive a child.

DIANE: So having a masculine identity doesn't necessarily mean they don't want to become pregnant? So how does that affect day-to-day business?

ALICE: Exactly. We're starting to train our staff—because we're a feminist organization—and now we're working to change the language on the rest of our website to "recipients and partners," instead of "single moms and lesbian couples." And also, we make sure we understand if someone prefers male pronouns, for example, we put it in their file so when our office has contact with them we use male pronouns. So those changes in language and identity are really important things we didn't used to think about as much.

DIANE: Why do you think trans people are coming forward to have children now, when they didn't used to?

ALICE: I think we're seeing this change because, historically, trans folks either didn't come out, or didn't feel comfortable engaging with the medical system in that way. When you become a parent you have to deal with not just your child, but with institutions in a way you never had to before. You're dealing with societal institutions in a different way, with schools, and pediatric departments, and childcare, and all this stuff. And when you're in a culture that is discriminatory, it can be very scary and unsafe, both for the parent and the child. And I think we're starting to see shifts culturally around that, and those shifts that are happening culturally are starting to appear in the fertility arena.

It's affected me personally as well. I used to say, when I was telling my son his conception story, that women have eggs and men have sperm and I needed sperm to have you so I asked my friend for his sperm and he said yes and that's how I had you. Now I say, most of the time the people who have sperm are men and the people who have eggs and a uterus are women, but not always, and look at all this diversity we have in our community.

And my son is growing up with a very different perspective than we have, because he's grown up with a teacher in his afterschool program who is nonbinary and uses the pronoun "they." And he has adults in his life who are out as trans people. And he has adults and children in his summer camp that are nonbinary. And he told me he tried out the pronoun "they" for a week in his summer camp because his friend did and he just wanted to see what it felt like.

I also have a relative who came out as nonbinary a little while ago and I told my son and he said, "Oh, so they don't feel like a she anymore. OK." And that was that. He has no problem with their pronoun. To me, the thing is to respect another person as a human being and call them what they want you to call them.

The evolution of TSBC's business corresponds directly to changes in the social environment, in which we see an expanded awareness of the range of people's experiences vis-à-vis their bodies, which do not necessarily correspond to the biological sex with which they were born. In addition, with gradually decreasing stigma, and increasing technological possibilities, trans people will have greater reproductive options, thereby creating new ways of thinking about people who carry a child and give birth. Not everyone who delivers a child from one's body identifies as a woman or a mother.

I asked Maya to help me understand the intersections between increased awareness of trans people and expanded reproductive technology options.

MAYA: When I first came out in high school in the eighties, I consciously felt like I couldn't be myself and be a parent at the same time, until I later met other lesbian and queer-identified parents. It was primarily lesbians and gays who were building families together. And I saw this film, *Choosing Children*, in 1985 and I thought, "Aha, if I'm able to have a child with my body I would love to do home insemination with a known donor." But from where I first began seeing a pathway to parenthood, it took me another nineteen years to see my way forward to having a baby.

It was a very different time on many fronts. We didn't have the language of "cis" and "trans" but it was primarily "cis" gay donors who most lesbians chose. At that time, queer folks and lesbians and gay folks and the LGBTQ community were really facing the loss of custody if they were to come out while parenting. So many people chose—because sperm banks weren't open to queer people—an anonymous donor for the sperm in order to protect their rights as parents. But I wanted to have conception with a known donor—someone who we would now call a cis gay male.

My partner is not someone who saw being masculine identified and pregnant as a positive thing, although a lot of folks do. So he wasn't really interested in getting pregnant and I was very interested in getting pregnant. So we took a class at MAIA Midwifery in 2001, around conception options for LGBTQ people, and wrote a letter to our community to find a Chinese Mexican, or Asian Latinx, HIV-negative donor.

So we wanted a tall, cis gay man, who was HIV negative. At the time, there was no information on how HIV-positive men could safely have children, but now they can because technology has advanced to make it safe. So, my partner wanted tall with good teeth. I focused on someone who was out to his family, who was a good communicator, and who was gay. And that's a really important part of sperm is that a lot of us are actually looking for a gay donor, or trans or gay sperm. Whether there's the nature-nurture aspect of it, especially since we're having known donors we wanted someone who was going to fit into our family.

It was also really important that whoever he was, our donor was out to their family so that we were not at risk for grandparents trying to take away parental rights. At the time, we were really concerned about that. And there were a lot of women in the lesbian community who were losing custody of their children. The laws in California protect us quite a bit now, but back then in 2000–2001, we took quite a risk.

Also at that time we also didn't see a lot of trans women being sperm donors. But now in the community you have people helping each other out. So somebody has eggs, somebody has sperm, somebody has embryos, and uteruses, and all of those parts don't necessarily belong to a woman's or a man's body. And I think the whole way in which we talk about reproduction has changed a lot. The book *What Makes a Baby*, by Cory Silverberg, visually depicts a radical paradigm shift in how babies come to be. Factually speaking, it takes a sperm, an egg, and a uterus in order to make conception happen, but whose bodies and what they call themselves can be really, really varied.

Maya's experience raises a number of important issues. First, for many people seeking parenthood outside a heterosexual relationship, the pathway to parenthood can be long and require substantially more planning and consideration than it does for straight couples. Second, while there have been some improvements for LGBTQ people, fears surrounding loss of custody—especially in the 1980s and 1990s—played a significant role in how people selected known sperm donors, as well as sperm bank donors. In addition, HIV-positive men are now able to contribute sperm to produce a child—either their own child or as a known donor—because technologies are available that separate sperm (which does not carry HIV) from the semen (which does). Third, there have been substantial changes regarding how we think about gender, the body, and reproduction, including linguistic shifts toward more inclusivity of different identities, as well as shifts toward breaking down conceptions of the body into different parts—eggs, sperm, wombs—that are not linked to gender or sexual identity. This nonbinary way of talking and thinking about identity and the body represents an enormous linguistic and cultural shift regarding how families are formed.

I asked Maya how these changes in thinking intersect with people's reproductive options. She responded,

There are huge shifts. Some organizations, like Our Family Coalition, bring together people looking for egg donors, sperm donors, and surrogates through an egg meets sperm networking mixer. I'm also seeing embryo donation within queer and trans families in the past five years. If people plan to get pregnant and would use a sperm donor, then they may look into using embryo donation instead of sperm and egg donation. From an economic standpoint that makes total sense. It's a lot cheaper.

I'm part of a Facebook group where this is happening, where people are considering egg donation, sperm donation, or embryo donation. Like me, I'm fifty-one, I can't use my own eggs but my uterus is healthy. If I were to pay for conception with an egg donor that's going to be about $26,000–$50,000.

And if I'm going to use a sperm donor on top of that it's another $800 to $1,000 per vial, and that's not even including the procedures. I just talked to someone two days ago who is doing home inseminations and it's costing her $800 per vial, out of pocket. You also have to pay an initiation fee on top of that. So some people work privately with reproductive endocrinologists who know people who have gone through IVF [in vitro fertilization] already, and who have a known relationship with recipients of their embryos. Some of those people who have embryos stored are deciding to donate them to other people, rather than use them or destroy them or donate them to science.

But most of the embryo donation programs are run by Christian organizations, and will only provide embryos for heterosexual married couples. If you're a single parent of any gender or sexual orientation, or queer, or don't fit into that heterosexual married scope, they're not going to provide you with embryos. People pretty much have to go through private doctors to get access. And a lot of them call it "embryo adoption" instead of embryo donation, which is language I find problematic.

I'm seeing a lot of people in their forties and fifties who have fertility challenges and are thinking about embryo donation. I would say there's a movement within the trans and queer communities and single-parent communities to open up known embryo donation—especially for people past their reproductive age.

For people attempting to conceive outside sexual intercourse or use low-tech procedures like home insemination, access to reproductive technologies is essential. For many, the cost can be prohibitive. Embryo donation combined with in vitro fertilization can be a slightly more affordable option than sperm or egg donation. A number of Christian organizations have launched embryo "adoption" agencies, in order to enable heterosexual couples with leftover frozen embryos from infertility treatments donate them to someone else, rather than destroy them or freeze them indefinitely (Cromer, 2017). These organizations, however, discuss embryos and babies as morally equivalent, have a political-religious agenda that many in the LGBTQ community are loath to associate with, and would not provide services to people outside the heteronormative family structure anyway.

Maya's story parallels that of another family I met in Los Angeles, at a conference for LGBTQ family-building options in 2016. Brenda was a thirty-five-year-old white woman who worked as a reproductive counselor. Her partner, Shawn, was a twenty-eight-year-old African American trans man. Together they have a son, five, from Shawn's brother's sperm. Because of Brenda's work, they have many connections in the community of people who want to help them have a second child. One of their friends is a thirty-year-old white trans man who went through the egg retrieval process to freeze his eggs before he transitioned. He produced a large number of eggs on his retrieval cycle and offered to share them with Shawn and Brenda to use with their donor. However, their donor, Shawn's brother, did not want to donate again because he had gotten married and his wife was opposed to it. Shawn and Brenda found another African American known donor through a network of friends, so they decided to create embryos with their friend's eggs. Brenda told me about their journey:

> Our friends tried first and they didn't get pregnant with their embryos. And that put us in a really sensitive place, ethically. We had gone through the legal paperwork and finished that process while they were going through the IVF process. They had frozen sperm and we had fresh sperm and they had many less viable embryos than we did. A lot of the embryos just didn't develop. By the end, we only had about three healthy embryos. We didn't feel right donating our embryos to them, because our sperm donor didn't know them. So they're just being stored.
>
> After that, I had some friends who went through IVF with an egg donor. They're both *really* white and they used a white egg donor. They have two children, and they had leftover embryos, and offered to donate their extra embryos to us. So we thought about that. But then we would be this mixed-race couple with a super-white baby, and we didn't know if it made sense to have this super-white baby in our mixed-race family and community, especially because everyone would question Shawn's relationship to the child, and he's already marginalized as a trans man of color.
>
> Another lesbian friend was willing to donate her eggs to us, but she was Brazilian and Japanese. Again being a family that is African American and white, the values for us would be if I carried a child who is genetically a mix of both of us. And of course our child would know the donor, but I don't know if I'm equipped to teach a child about Japanese and Brazilian culture. So there's all these things to consider. It's really complicated.

Brenda's quandary regarding choosing sperm, eggs, or embryos that fit her family constellation illustrates another element of grassroots eugenics. Her personal values surrounding community, family, partnership, and genetic perceptions inform her decisions concerning what her potential future child might look and be like. Grassroots eugenics turns traditional eugenics on its head in a way that is contrary to the mainstream. It is a type of reproductive activism, an attempt to create people who are more open-minded, more inclusive, and more intersectional. Brenda and her partner question what it means to belong to their family.

For example, could they offer an Brazilian Japanese African American child enough of the child's Brazilian Japanese heritage in a multiracial family of a different composition—especially given that they have one child who is biologically related to both parents? How would having a white child with no apparent mixed ancestry fit both with Brenda's partner—whose connection to his child is already questioned—and with the ethnic mix of her existing family? Sexuality also comes into play: for a variety of reasons, having a trans or gay known sperm donor fits better with her family and community than a heterosexual donor.

These stories reveal the complexities of planning a family outside a heterosexual relationship, as well as the different possible constellations of family creation—both technologically and socially. Brenda and those close to her pursued various combinations of egg, sperm, and embryo donation. Involving transfers from one body to another through clinical intersections and across blurred distinctions of race, sex, and gender, her experience encapsulates the range of possibilities for family creation via technology.

Maya's and Brenda's journeys to parenthood led them through a range of technological possibilities, with resourceful ways of making and defining family. I asked Maya how she defines family. She responded, "My brother has a beautiful frame for it, he says, 'We're not a nuclear family, we're a "molecular family."' We're pulled together through some mysterious chemistry. I love the image of that. We're these different molecules that are all connected, and come together, and have these different formations that draws us together."

DONOR CONCEPTION AND MOLECULAR FAMILIES

Maya's brother's term, "molecular family," provides a useful frame for thinking about donor-conceived family relationships, extended family, and broader social-familial networks beyond the nuclear family structure. Donor-conceived families have a range of biological and social compositions, varying degrees of connection and openness between the donor and the donor-conceived child, and new kin terminologies to reflect new formations of genetic and familial ties. Up until 2004, when the Ethics Committee of the American Society for Reproductive Medicine (Ethics Committee of the ASRM 2004) published an opinion in favor of openness—stating that children should be told how they were conceived—the norm for clinics and businesses providing eggs and sperm was anonymity and secrecy. If a parent plans to tell his or her child that the child was donor conceived, the child may want to have more information about the donor who provided the genetic material that helped create him or her, whether out sheer curiosity or for medical history.

Since its inception, TSBC has offered identity-release donors and has offered donor-conceived children their identity-release donor's contact information once the child reaches eighteen. For years, it was the only sperm bank to do so. By the time I revisited TSBC in 2017, they had done away with their anonymous donor program the year prior and only offered identity-release donors. I asked Alice why they stopped offering anonymous donation. She explained,

> The vast majority of parents plan to tell their children how they were conceived. And the vast majority of parents choose identity-release donors. When I got here, about 60 percent or more of our donors were identity release, and 80 percent of sales were in the ID-release program. The non-identity-release donors just weren't selling well.
>
> And we've had some donors who wanted to be anonymous actually end up being identified. Since these DNA databases have emerged, and 23 and Me and Ancestry.com, some have been found that way. That's happened other places too. We felt like we couldn't promise the donors anonymity. We didn't feel good about that for donors who didn't want to be identified. It's now too likely that they'll be discovered. So I want donors who know that and will be OK with that.

Advances in genetic testing, DNA technologies, and databases enable donor-conceived offspring (as well as adoptees) to find each other. The Donor Sibling Registry allows donor-conceived people to connect with their donors and children of the same donor, as well as enabling donor-conceived families to connect with one another. An array of other groups launched by donor-conceived adults and their allies—such as donorchildren.com, wearedonorconceived.com, and dnadectectives.com—also help donor-connected people find biological kin through genetic test kits, ancestry sleuthing, and facilitating online forum.

When I first visited TSBC years ago, none of the children conceived from their donors had yet turned eighteen. The first child to turn eighteen after they opened for business did so in 2001. According to Alice at TSBC, approximately 70 percent or more of heterosexual clients tell their children they were donor conceived, and all of the single women and lesbian couples did. Since Alice came on board in 2002, many children have come forward to get information about their donors, and Alice has been in charge of facilitating those connections. She has been researching how donor-conceived children request contact with their donors.

> We thought more people would come forward. It's only about 30 percent. Most are between eighteen and twenty. We did phone interviews and a questionnaire. What I find is they have very low expectations. I don't know if they're suppressing their feelings because they don't want to get their hopes up. But they say things like, "Well you know I've always been curious and I just want to know if he looks like me. And if he just wants to provide a picture, that's OK."
>
> So I have a conversation with them about their expectations and how to manage them. Sometimes we think we don't have any assumptions or expectations until those aren't met. So I have a conversation with them about possible mismatched

expectations. The best outcomes are where people have matched goals and expectations. It's not about how much contact they have, it's whether they're satisfied with the contact they have.

TSBC also offers families who share donors the opportunity to connect with one another. About 30 percent of TSBC clients request contact with other families who used the same donor. Alice continued,

We don't necessarily think genetics equals family, or that people from the same donor are siblings and they have a right to know them. Our approach is that some people are interested in these relationships, some people aren't. But if people want to be in contact with each other we will help facilitate that. Sometimes when they're a little older and their kid takes a high school biology class they come home and say, "I just realized there might be other kids from my donor. Can I meet them?"

Our intention is to put people who share a donor in contact with each other. What those families are to each other is up to them. So some of those people consider each other family and may consider those children siblings to their children. They may consider those families special friends and their children special friends, or they may consider them something in between. I've heard "dibling" from the donor sibling registry. I've heard our families use "dosi," like short for "donor sibling," cute for small children. But donors are donors, not biological fathers. Parents are parents, regardless of whether or not they are biologically connected to their children.

Language has changed to accommodate new social and biological relationships engineered by assisted reproductive technologies. These reflect nonbiological parents' status, how donors are perceived and categorized, the relationship between donor-conceived children, and even donor perceptions of the children conceived via their egg or sperm donation. In my current research, egg donors commonly refer to the children born from their eggs as their "egg babies"—not their children but still connected. Families linked through donor-conceived children may consider themselves family or may not.

So who seeks out other families conceived from the same donor? Heterosexual couples rarely want to connect with other donor-conceived families. The majority of these couples live in a nuclear family structure, where the family includes the mother, the father, and their children—regardless of how they were conceived—and some of them have not told their children they were conceived with a sperm donor. Lesbian couples often have an extensive social network of other moms with donor-conceived kids. According to Alice, single women— especially single, heterosexual women—reach out the most to connect with other families, looking for community:

The single moms, by definition, have smaller families because they're only one parent, and it can be very isolating. They're not as likely to have community of other single moms. When I was trying to conceive, I had many other lesbian friends who were trying to conceive at the same time.

I think as a group, single heterosexual women come from a more traditional perspective and think shared genetics makes a sibling. Whereas some lesbian couples feel that way and some don't.

Because many people in the queer community have to let go of biological family, they form friendship families. There's a broader understanding of kinship and what that means.

This difference between how single, heterosexual women and lesbian and bisexual women perceive family, kinship, and connectedness is profound. Alice's observations resonate both with what I have seen throughout this research, in talking to other women in a range of family configurations, and with my own experiences of isolation and struggle as a single mother clinging to a nuclear family mind-set.

Existing research demonstrates that children born into families with two parents—regardless of the parents' sexual orientation—fare better than do children raised in single-parent families. As Susan Golombok (2015) points out, this is due not to any deficiencies on the part of single mothers per se but rather to a broader lack of support, financial vulnerability, a lack of social connectedness, and the difficulty of managing all the responsibilities of child-rearing and subsistence on one's own. She writes that the large body of research on psychological difficulties facing children of single-mother families can be accounted for by the "adverse factors that commonly accompany single parenthood . . . including economic hardship, maternal depression and lack of social support" (2015, 196). For single-parent families, the nuclear model does not work, and for most single parents, the "molecular family model" does not appear as a possibility. As Maya stated, "I feel like the nuclear family is inadequate for most folks. I'm happy to put that model to bed."

CONCLUSION

There have been substantial social and technological changes surrounding parenthood and family creation over the past twenty years; in many ways, these changes are interconnected. Changing definitions of family, increased legal protection for same-sex marriage, and advances in reproductive technologies provide people with more stability, access to health insurance benefits, recognition as next of kin, and procreation options. While same-sex marriage is federally recognized, protections for children born into same-sex unions and parental rights to the children produced in those relationships vary from state to state. California has been at the forefront of recognizing same-sex partnerships, and the rights of parents and children in families formed from those partnerships, but this has not been without the sustained efforts of political activists to change the law in order to meet LGBTQ family needs. This chapter has addressed some of the shifts in thinking that have occurred regarding family and family creation through technologies, but this overview is by no means exhaustive.

Marriage equality and advances in technology have affected the reproductive technology industry. Newer technologies, such as intracytoplasmic sperm injection, virtually eliminated heterosexual couples as clients in the sperm-banking industry. Sperm banks opened their services to all people, regardless of marital status, gender, or sexual orientation. They could no longer afford to discriminate against those who fell outside the realm of married, male-female couples. With legal recognition of same-sex marriage in California, TSBC began to see lesbian couples coming in to start their families earlier. Not only did their efforts change California law, but they also had a direct impact at the federal level, altering the language used by the FDA. These regulatory changes created increased access to medical treatment, as the medical providers were no longer required to uphold discriminatory laws. The shift in the ASRM's position on providing access enhanced people's reproductive options. Some physicians and clinics may still deny same-sex couples or single people access, but this would be more due to their own personal beliefs and prejudices rather than legal barriers.

Some of the most significant changes over the past twenty-plus years have had to do with the options available for same-sex male couples. As Leland noted, in his generation, gay men rarely considered becoming parents—and far less often than lesbians. While lesbian women faced many challenges, it was far easier and more affordable for them to get sperm than it was for men to have access to donor eggs and surrogacy. In the early 2000s, gay men began to adopt from abroad. For same-sex male couples with financial resources, though, egg donation and surrogacy became preferred avenues once international adoption options began to decrease.

Through grassroots organizing and activism, Leland and Maya worked to expand existing laws defining *sexually intimate partners* to include women who were using known sperm donors to do home inseminations. While regulatory blockades prohibiting access to advanced reproductive technologies may exist, people who need these services either figure out their way around the law—by finding LGBT-friendly medical practitioners—or work to change the law.

Third-party reproduction through gamete donation and surrogacy further transformed the definitions of family and required new language to address new biological and social relationships. A person may be biologically, socially, or gestationally a mother, or all of the above, and genetic lineage can be separate from parenting and caring (Cahn and Carbone 2003). A person who provided sperm may be a father, a donor, an "uncle," or a "special friend." These categories change according to the social role one occupies. Genetics no longer determine family. Notions of sex and gender have expanded beyond binary categories. The range of family and gender identities can best be thought of as a spectrum of meanings and identities, rather than predetermined codes based in binary, biological sex.

10 · CONCLUSION
Toward a New BioPoliTechs
of Emerging Families

Much has changed over the past two decades in regard to family formation via technology. My examination of the interplay between assisted reproductive technologies, the people who use them, those who provide reproductive products and services—with the overarching legal, political, social, and medical institutions—explores the range of negotiations, conformities, and rebellions involved in creating and recognizing family. Throughout this work, I have thought in terms of intersections, collages, and spectrums, rather than boundaries and false binary categories.

There have been significant changes in the overall acceptance of same-sex parents and single people having children with donor gametes and other forms of third-party reproduction. These changes are evident in shifts in language and medical practice, increased legal recognition of same-sex marriages, and increased social acceptance of the range of family forms. One of the most significant changes is an increased awareness about transgender identities and reproductive needs.

Language has evolved to be more inclusive of a range of identities and, in relation to that, cultural perceptions of what it means to human and gendered have broadened. This takes us back to the Sapir-Whorf hypothesis to some degree: language can influence, and perhaps shape, our interpretation of the world around us (Whorf 1956; Sapir 1961), but evolving perceptions of that world may also influence changes in language. This is certainly true with expanded, nonbinary gendered definitions and thinking about the body and gender as not necessarily correlated with biological sex.

Legal definitions of family have broadened significantly. With the passage of *Obergefell v. Hodges*, same-sex marriage is now legally recognized in the United States at the national level.[1] While *Obergefell* did not speak specifically to the presumption of parentage, and LGBTQ family and custody protections vary from state to state, there is already evidence of change on this front as well. Since

Obergefell, there have already been new cases speaking directly to the rights of LGBTQ people to have their families recognized and to have both parents listed on the birth certificate. In *Pavan v. Smith*, the U.S. Supreme Court rejected the Arkansas Supreme Court's ruling that certain "biological truths" prevented two mothers from being recognized as their child's parents on the birth certificate.[2] These decisions will likely lead to more states recognizing LGBTQ families, as well as more legal challenges for people to have their families legally protected.

Some of the most significant changes pertain to expanded reproductive technological possibilities. The reproductive technology industry has grown exponentially since I first started this research. In the 1990s, donor insemination among single women and two-mother families was becoming increasingly common. Single women preferred the sperm bank option over remaining childless because they could not find a partner. The rise of HIV/AIDS led more lesbian and bisexual women to use sperm banks rather than known donors, but many still preferred a donor they knew. Sperm banks also offered two-mom families better legal protection than they could secure by using known donors. While other technologies, like *in vitro* fertilization, egg donation, and surrogacy, certainly were available for heterosexual couples, it was not common for same-sex male couples to use these options at the time. For men who did want to parent, some pursued adoption— especially international adoption—until international adoption started becoming less accessible for them. Some gay and bisexual men saw known sperm donation as one avenue toward at least having some contact with a child born from their sperm.

In the early 2000s, access to assisted reproductive technologies began to expand, and more men started thinking about having their own biological families, rather than forming a relationship with a child either as a known donor or through adoption. Men's use of assisted reproductive technologies increased as adoption options shut down. Male same-sex couples, however, need both an egg and someone to carry and deliver their child. Some, like Leland and his partner, used traditional surrogates—a woman who was directly inseminated with the intended father's sperm and using her own egg, through a process called intrauterine insemination (IUI). At the time, traditional surrogacy was more common than gestational surrogacy. In gestational surrogacy, a donor egg is fertilized in vitro—known as *in vitro* fertilization (IVF)—and then the embryo is transferred to the surrogate. Gestational surrogacy is far more costly and a more medically invasive process for both the surrogate and the egg donor. Traditional surrogacy is less expensive for intended parents, it is an easier process for the surrogate, and it avoids the need for a separate egg donor. Most fertility clinics now provide only gestational surrogacy services, as traditional surrogacy is deemed too legally and emotionally risky: if a surrogate carries her biological child—who contractually belongs to someone else—she may have a greater tendency to be emotionally attached to the child she delivers and challenge the surrogacy contract in court.

In the 1990s men who did not have female partners but wanted children had limited options, and people who were HIV positive faced imminent death, so having a child was unlikely. Now, with antiretroviral therapy, HIV/AIDS is a chronic disease a person can live with for decades. Because HIV/AIDS is no longer an immediate death sentence, many HIV-positive people want to have children. With new information about how HIV/AIDS is transmitted, HIV-positive men are able to become parents, due to improved sperm-washing techniques that separate sperm from semen. Fertility practices have adjusted or emerged to meet the growing demand of men wanting babies. Some, like *Growing Generations*, specifically cater to same-sex male partners, single men, and HIV-positive men, offering egg donation and surrogacy services.

This growing demand for gestational surrogates and egg donors to meet the reproductive needs of single men and same-sex male couples—as well as others who use egg donation and surrogacy—presents an array of ethical dilemmas that having a child via sperm donation does not. Sperm donation carries no risk to the donor. However, egg donation exposes donors to potentially harmful hormones and surgery under anesthesia, and any pregnancy—whether as a surrogate or for one's own child—carries risk. In both cases, these risks are understudied and many have called for more research in this area (Beeson and Lippman 2006; Schneider, Lahl, and Kramer 2017). This raises concerns as to whether women who provide these services for pay are being exploited, and to what degree financial compensation for those who are economically vulnerable may cloud informed consent.

In my exploration of agency and subversion in response to discrimination and exclusion, I have asked, How does the use of reproductive technologies both conform to and upend societal standards and stigmas, as well as lead to reformulations and reconstitutions of family, beyond both social and biological categories? Technologies are not created in a social vacuum, nor does society exist in a technological vacuum. They intersect and transform each other, and ultimately lead to new ways of thinking and new questions: What underlying assumptions and drives influence technological creation and innovation in the first place? How does social change influence how technologies are used and who has access to them? How do the actual uses of technologies evolve from the initial intention of their use? For example, assisted reproductive technologies emerged with the intent of enabling infertile women—assumed to be heterosexual and married—to bear children. They were not intended for single people and same-sex couples, and they were not developed to help trans people preserve fertility or reproduce. But although single people, same-sex couples, and especially trans people once faced enormous obstacles in getting access to reproductive technologies, once technologies are made available, people will find a way to access them—despite the obstacles. With time, the obstacles break down completely.

Since I first started this work, the social-political-technological trends have changed, same-sex couples can now get married, and the tide has shifted toward legally recognizing the families they create—somewhat. With the U.S. Supreme Court's recognition of same-sex couples' right to marry, it follows that children would be part of that. The battles over the parental rights of same-sex couples and nonbiological partners are still being waged, and laws vary from state to state.

BIOPOLITECHS AND THE HUMAN FUTURE

Many researchers have explored assisted reproduction, family formation, and family planning, drawing on Foucauldian notions of biopolitics and power, of the regulation and management of life, and how institutions subjugate and control political subjects, populations, and reproductive bodies (Scheper-Hughes 2002, 2007; Davis-Floyd 2004; L. Cohen 2004; Waldby and Cooper 2008; Towghi 2013; Mills 2006; Inhorn 2007a; Ong and Collier 2008; Krause and de Zordo 2012; de Zordo and Marchesi 2015; Varley 2012). In writing this book I have begun to consider: Is there something specific about how reproductive technologies are accessed and used within the biopolitical framework? Is it worthwhile to think in terms of "biopolitechs"—to explore the specific intersections between biopolitics, biopower, and reproductive and biotechnologies and the creation of varied forms of life?

In much of Foucault's work he addresses how individual subjects self regulate in response to external technologies of power, observation, and domination, in order to attain a state of happiness and acceptance, or to avoid isolation, punishment, or torture (Foucault 1975, 1988). Here, technologies of power are external, they objectivize the subject, and the subject makes internal adjustments to adapt and conform. It seems to me, however, that there is something unique about technological reproduction and biotechnological innovation that is different from other examples of how technologies intersect with biopower and biopolitics. From genes, to genetic testing and diagnosis and DNA databases (Benjamin 2013), to the creation of new forms of human beings through genetic manipulation, to reproductive labor, to cyborg humans and hybrid animal chimeras (Haraway 1991, 1997)—all of these phenomena are connected to and created within biopolitical systems, emanating from sets of assumptions about the body, economic and social value, gender, race and class, and a desire to manipulate the future of life. It is essential to examine these interactions and intersections, individual and social conformities and disruptions, and the potential for both future transformations and intensified inequalities as they relate to bio- and repro-technological development.

Reproductive technologies are embodied technologies and, as such, they are internalized and transformed. While broader biopolitical constraints do regulate who has access to them, and work to maintain mainstream social norms, the individual drive to have a child calls for resistance against those norms and can result in transforming society, rather than necessarily being controlled by it. The individual is not a passive responder to external social controls. Foucault, himself, comes closer to the notion of individual agency, when he states: "Perhaps I've insisted too much in the technology of domination and power. I am more and more interested in the interaction between oneself and in the technologies of individual domination, the history of how an individual acts upon himself, in the technology of the self" (Foucault 1988, 18). Technologies can be used both to maintain and subvert the dominant system, but once created—in part because they intersect with humans who adapt technologies to their own needs—they cannot be contained. Of course, not to forget, that social inequality and financial security create a hierarchy of access to these technologies.

When I first started this research years ago, I was interested in how lay perceptions of genetics—what I call "folk genetics"—influence donor choice. I reasoned that women choosing donors without having to match the donor to a male partner might provide greater insight into how people make meaning out of genetic material. I was partially right; although, most lesbian couples wanted to physically match the donor to their female partner, and most single women wanted a donor with the physical characteristics of someone they would be attracted to. Selecting for social characteristics was more complicated for both groups.

Thomas Kuhn's (1963) classic book *The Structure of Scientific Revolutions* demonstrates how scientific paradigms shift over time and, after some rejection, resistance, and gradual acceptance, new paradigms replace old ones. This is no less true for geneticists' understandings of how genetic inheritance works. Folk genetic understandings influence reproductive behavior. At the level of the state and through medical and social policy, "positive" eugenic programs attempt to enhance the reproduction of some groups over others through pronatalist policies for some and family-planning promotion for others. These practices are rooted in the belief that some people have more intrinsic value than others—a genetic belief system infused with racist, classist, and heteronormative assumptions.

Popular perceptions of genetics influence both reproductive behavior and scientific practice. In the process of selecting donors, most intended parents have a list of criteria that their donor must meet, much of which has nothing at all to do with genetic heritability at the biological level. What I call grassroots eugenics is when people choose donors according to their own idiosyncratic beliefs surrounding genetic and social value. These perceptions are variable, personal, and connected to individuals' assessments of the people and community they want to create and the world they want to live in.

Another level of analysis concerns how some people become the providers of reproductive products and labor within the broader biotechnological and reproductive market. Whether providing clinical labor as a research subject (Cooper and Waldby 2014) or providing goods and services for pay as a reproductive worker (Tober 2002; Tober and Pavone 2018) the people who offer parts of their bodies to others usually share a common denominator: financial need. Gamete providers and gestational surrogates do want to help other people who are struggling to have a family, but the majority would not do it if it were not for the compensation—especially when it comes to the more physically intrusive and riskier terrain of female reproductive labor. Indeed, the discourses of female reproductive labor vacillate between feminine power and exploitation (Roberts 1998). Sperm provision, on the other hand, does not raise these same concerns.

Compensation is not necessarily a bad thing. For egg providers and gestational surrogates, the risk of complications—whether from fertility drugs, medical procedures, or gestation, labor, and delivery—is substantially higher. In my current research with U.S. and international egg providers, many women express the joy they experience when they find out they helped someone else have a baby. On the other hand, there are a substantial number of women in my study—which consists of over ninety interviews and almost two hundred surveys to date—who have experienced major health complications either directly related or possibly related to the drugs and procedures.[3] In the international market for human eggs, many donors report feeling as though they are treated as "egg machines" instead of patients. This raises serious concerns regarding the commodification of the body, how economic inequalities drive decision making, the impact on people who provide reproductive services, and the lack of regulation of a booming international fertility market in which eggs are golden (Tober and Pavone 2018).

New technologies create new possibilities. But they also create new concerns and present a range of ethical quandaries specific to technology and power (L. Cohen 2008; Scheper-Hughes, 2002). Some people have the financial wherewithal to access technologies, whether in the United States or abroad. Many go on fertility-seeking holidays, whether for *in vitro* fertilization to conceive and carry their own biological children, or with local or foreign egg providers (Speier 2016). As the demand for cross-border fertility care rises, so, too, does the demand for female bioavailable bodies to provide these egg products and gestational services (Nahman 2016).[4]

Egg donation and surrogacy spark international debates on what it means to be a mother. Single women and same-sex female couples can use donor sperm to have a child. However, men do not have access to surrogacy, leading many same-sex Spanish male couples to seek surrogates in the United States, particularly California, or other international destinations. In Spain, legally, the mother of the child is the one who gives birth to it. This is the case in many countries, leading to new challenges for people pursuing international surrogacy and egg donation options. There are also many cases, due to conflicting and inconsistent international laws, in which children born from surrogacy arrangements in other countries have been left stateless. The ethical quandaries for international surrogacy have many parallels to those presented by international adoption (Scherman et al. 2016). Many countries that were global hotspots for reproductive tourism—for example, India and Thailand, and others—have shut their doors to those seeking such services, while other countries simultaneously emerge to pick up the slack.

There are always new technologies on the horizon. A recent advance in egg-freezing technology, a process of flash-freezing called vitrification, now enables women to freeze their eggs when they are younger in case they need to use them in the future. Perhaps egg-freezing technologies will offer new possibilities to women who want to develop their careers, wait for the right partner, or just wait until they are ready to have a child so that they can create their family on their own terms (Benintendi 2017; Lehman-Haupt 2016; Richards 2013). Perhaps egg freezing would have helped some of the women in my study who faced their own age-related infertility due to "old eggs." But the quest for a technological fix seems easier than challenging corporate culture to accommodate all parents with family-friendly policies (Tober 2018). While an exciting possibility for reproductive freedom, we do not yet know whether egg freezing will indeed turn out to be the fertility-preserving insurance policy that people—including both women and trans men—hope for, or whether it will present a new collection of techno-logical coercions and social and emotional challenges.

Other new reproductive technologies that are just coming to the fore include those that create what have been commonly called "three-parent babies" through mitochondrial DNA (mtDNA) replacement. This process was first made legal in the United Kingdom in 2015 as a way to prevent the transmission of mitochon-drial disease to one's offspring. The process involves extracting the diseased mtDNA from the intended mother's egg and replacing it with healthy mtDNA from a donor egg. The new egg is then fertilized with a sperm cell, and after the embryo develops into a blastocyst, it is transferred to a recipient—either the intended mother or a gestational surrogate—to carry. This process would cre-ate a child that carries the nuclear DNA of the intended mother and the mtDNA of the egg donor, but the resulting child would resemble the intended mother. Ethical concerns regarding this technique center on the "slippery slope," and the unknown consequences, of permanent human germline engineering (Baylis 2013; Darnovsky 2013; Obasogie and Darnovsky 2018). Same-sex couples also hold out hope that, one day soon, assisted reproductive technologies will be able to create embryos with two eggs or two sperm, so couples can have their own biological child, with both partners contributing equally.

Throughout this book I have explored the intersections between access to and use of reproductive technologies, the reproductive industry, overarching governmental regulations, societal expectations and settings, the donors who provide sperm as a product, and the people who purchase it or access it to create their families. Emerging technologies, reproductive and otherwise, are changing the human present and the human future. These are not only important anthropological and social science concerns but are also of enormous relevance to society at large. For people who are connected through third-party reproduction— whether donors, intended parents, donor-conceived children, or practitioners in the fertility industry—relevance goes beyond academic debates to lived, embodied experiences. By following the course of assisted reproduction and family creation and recognition from the 1990s to today, I have demonstrated in this book how quickly technology and culture evolve and move together, toward as yet unimagined futures.

AFTERWORD

Aside from my professional journey through this project as an anthropologist, this has also been a personal journey. Through my own experiences as a single mother, which has at times been both arduous and rewarding, I often reflected on women's stories and how they related to my own life. People I spoke to for this book showed me possibilities I had never thought of, especially in terms of living life on my own terms, thinking about family, and thinking beyond isolating nuclear limitations and toward more communal, "molecular" linkages. We often think of anthropologists as professionals who go out into the field, study something, and objectively report back. This has not been my experience. As a human being, I have had my own personal struggles. How I approached my work and the kinds of questions I asked were largely informed by my experiences. For me, fieldwork is also a transformative process. I see every person who took the time to speak with me as a gift, for which I am forever grateful. I hope this book does them justice.

ACKNOWLEDGMENTS

The research and writing of this book has been both a professional and a personal journey. The research would not have been possible if it had not been for the participation of the sperm bank professionals at the now-closed Repository for Germinal Choice, Leland Trainman at Rainbow Flag Health Services, and Barbara Raboy, Alice Ruby, Joanna Scheib and staff at The Sperm Bank of California, as well as other sperm banks and clinics I visited throughout this research. Thank you for opening your doors to me. I am extremely grateful to all the people who took the time to share their stories with me. They provided me with an enormous gift. They taught me to see possibilities I had never thought of before—especially in regard to living life on one's own terms. I hope this book does them justice.

Pursuing graduate training at the University of California, Berkeley/University of California, San Francisco, joint program in medical anthropology was a dream come true. Medical anthropologist Gay Becker first introduced me to the topic of infertility in 1989. I worked for Gay as a research assistant on her National Institutes of Health–funded research project exploring gender differences in response to infertility at the University of California, San Francisco. Gay's work set the methodological foundation for my own. I am forever grateful for her guidance and encouragement to explore this topic. Gay was on my mind every single day as I wrote this book. We lost her far too soon.

Nancy Scheper-Hughes was a mentor throughout my graduate training and has been a friend since. I am consistently inspired by her passion, energy, and persistence in the fight for human rights and social justice through activist anthropology. Her work on the commodification of the body and the black market in human organs influenced my thinking about the commodity quality of sperm. Lawrence Cohen, my postdoctoral mentor, also provided me with enormous support and guidance as I ventured into LGBTQ family formation, sperm donation, and sexuality research. Many others offered helpful comments and suggestions on earlier drafts, including other members of my committee Kristin Luker and Laura Nader; Stanley Brandes, who led a number of writing seminars; and my Berkeley cohort and colleagues—Vincanne Adams, David Eaton, Sandra Hyde, Kathleen Irwin, Peta Katz, Misha Klein, Elizabeth Roberts, and Kimberly Theidon, among others. Glenn Shepard deserves particular mention. When I presented my chapter on fantasy donors to the group, Glenn blurted out, "Oh, that's kind of like 'Romancing the Sperm.'" We all laughed, but the catchy title stuck. Thanks, Glenn.

This work would not have been possible without the generous support from the Social Science Research Council Sexuality Research Fellowship Program (SSRC/SRFP), with funds provided by the Ford Foundation. The two-year SRFP fellowship enabled me to add research on sperm donors to the project. Diane di Mauro was an eternally gracious and supportive SSCR/SRFP mentor and was delightful to spend time with at our many conferences and retreats. My co-fellows, Kate Frank and filmmaker-scholar Celine Parreñas Shimizu, among others SRFP scholars, provided ongoing inspiration and valuable feedback on my work. I am humbled and grateful for those on the selection committee who determined this project was worthy of funding.

While writing the current version of this book, I was a 2016–2017 Women's Policy Institute fellow, through the Women's Foundation of California. My Women's Policy Institute experience was exactly what I needed to expand my thinking regarding gender, sexuality, reproduction, and transgender issues, as well as the intersections between policy, individual action, and organizational advocacy. The program's director, Marj Plumb, worked tirelessly to not only educate about policy but also to raise awareness about how to be a better human being in an ever-complicated world. My experience as part of a reproductive justice team—and especially the inclusion of transgender people in the program—significantly contributed to the later chapters of this book. I am forever enriched by this experience.

Colleagues and staff at the University of California, San Francisco, Institute for Health and Aging, including Wendy Max and Regina Gudelunas, among others, provided me with intellectual care, sustenance, and an academic home. Barbara Koenig and Sharon Kaufman encouraged my re-entry into academia after many years in the nonprofit sector, to continue my research. My research assistants and interns, including Allyn Benintendi, Rella Kautiainan, Joanna Lamstein, and Meghna Mukherjee all kept my egg donor research project in forward motion while I was working on this book. Our regular conversations have been a constant source of intellectual stimulation.

I am eternally grateful for my editor at Rutgers University Press, Kimberly Guinta, for being such an enthusiastic and staunch supporter of this work. Jill Swenson, of Swenson Book Development, graciously held my hand through the writing process and gave me confidence in my writing and ideas when I did not have any. I am thankful for her edits on chapter drafts. I am also grateful to the anonymous reviewers, whose expertise and comments helped make this book better.

My friends and family have contributed in countless ways. My friend Maya Scott-Chung painstakingly read through my manuscript and helped me make new connections to explore current trends in LGBTQ family formation through assisted reproductive technologies. My friends Rachel Chadwell, Barbara Poratta, Leila Radan, Teri Thompson, and Lale Welsh have been by my side through the many years over which this project has unfolded and have supplied me with laughter and both healthy and unhealthy diversions. And of course, none of this would have been possible if it were not for the love and support of my family, who have stood by me through thick and thin. My brother Eric Tober and sister-in-law Elena Konstantinova-Tober may now live far away, but they always believe in me. My sons, Hunter and Tucker Durnford, were born around the same time I first started this work; they are my children, friends, and champions and have enriched my life beyond belief. My utmost gratitude goes to my parents, Lana and Bob Tober, who have supported me in all my hobbies and endeavors. Without your unwavering love and encouragement, none of this would have been possible.

NOTES

CHAPTER 1   MURPHY BROWN AND THE LESBIAN BABY BOOM

1. Dan Quayle's speech at the Commonwealth Club, "On Family Values," in San Francisco, CA, May 19, 1992. This address is commonly known as "The Murphy Brown Speech" for its reference to the television sit-com single working mother, Murphy Brown. http://www.vicepresidentdanquayle.com/speeches_StandingFirm_CCC_1.html

2. Mike Pence, speech delivered to the Republican Senate Committee in support of a constitutional amendment that would have defined marriage as between a man and a woman. 152 Cong. Rec. 14796 (2006).

3. Single Mothers by Choice is an organization that was founded by Jane Mattes in 1981. For Mattes, "single mothers by choice" refers to women who start out raising a child without a partner. This narrow definition excludes a range of people who end up parenting alone and does not address the range of people's experiences or the complexity of decision-making on the path to motherhood. See https://www.singlemothersbychoice.org. There is also a book by the same name (Mattes 1994).

CHAPTER 2   TECHNOLOGIES AND POLITICS OF REPRODUCTION

1. Human Fertilisation and Embryology Act, 1990, c. 37 (Eng.); Children Act, 1989, c. 41 (Eng.).

2. Human Fertilisation and Embryology Act, 2008, c. 22 (Eng.).

3. Rainbow Flag Health Services closed for business in 2012.

CHAPTER 3   SEMEN TO GO

1. Crandall v. Wagner, 71 Cal. App. 4th 724 (1999).

2. K.M. v. E.G., 37 Cal. 4th 130 (2005).

CHAPTER 4   SEMEN TRANSACTIONS

1. When I first interviewed Leland in 1999, he could only serve the San Francisco Bay Area. In the early 2000s he began shipping semen to many other states and had built an online clientele.

2. Masturbation Paradise, last accessed July 2001, http://www.masturbationparadise.com/banks.shtml (site discontinued).

CHAPTER 6   SEMEN AS GIFT, SEMEN AS GOODS

1. Johnson v. Superior Court (California Cryobank, Inc.), 101 Cal. App. 4th 869 (2002).

CHAPTER 7   FROM OLD "EGGS" TO "ODYSSEUS'S JOURNEY"

1. I want to emphasize that at the time of this research, and in the group of people I interviewed who were trying to conceive, all the people who were trying to get pregnant identified as women. At the time, the distinctions between cis women, trans women and transmasculine individuals were not being used, and none of the people trying to get pregnant identified as men. It is only more recently, as I will discuss in chapter 9, that trans men have been attempting to achieve pregnancy through donor insemination.

2. In IUIs, the semen is first washed to separate the sperm from the semen that contains it. If the sperm is not washed, the prostaglandins contained in the semen can cause uterine cramping and pain. The sperm is then injected into the uterus with a catheter.

3. GIFT, or gamete intrafallopian transfer, is a fertility treatment that involves removing the eggs, or mature oocytes, from a woman's ovaries via laparoscopy and putting both the egg and the sperm directly into the woman's fallopian tubes, allowing fertilization to take place in the uterus. For this process, the patient must take fertility drugs for several weeks in order to increase the number of eggs she produces (known as ovarian hyperstimulation). The physician measures her follicles throughout the process to determine when they are mature enough to administer a "trigger shot" of Lupron, HCG (human chorionic gonadotropin), or a mixture of both. About thirty-six hours later, the eggs are retrieved with an ultrasound-guided laparoscope. This procedure for retrieving oocytes is also used for IVF. But with IVF, the eggs are fertilized outside the body, in a petri dish, and then the embryo is transferred directly to the uterus.

4. DES is a nonsynthetic hormone that was given to pregnant women in order to help prevent miscarriage. Many women I have spoken to over the years who had problems with infertility were DES daughters. Between 1941 and 1971, approximately three million women were prescribed DES in the United States. Daughters born of mothers who took DES during pregnancy can have a range of fertility-related problems, including a T-shaped, or tipped, uterus; vaginal clear-cell adenocarcinomas; and other vaginal or cervical abnormalities. See, for example, Herbst, Ulfelder, and Poskanzer (1971).

CHAPTER 9   FROM MURPHY BROWN TO MODERN FAMILIES

1. Obergefell v. Hodges, 576 U.S. (2015), https://supreme.justia.com/cases/federal/us/576/14-556/opinion3.html.

2. Proposition 8 was a statewide ballot proposition in California that would have eliminated the rights of same-sex couples to marry. Opponents of same-sex marriage created it. California voters approved the measure in November 2008, making same-sex marriage illegal in California. On August 4, 2010, U.S. District chief judge Vaughn Walker overturned Proposition 8, stating that it "is unconstitutional under the Due Process Clause" and that the state has no interest that justifies denying same-sex couples the right to marry. See Brief of the American Psychological Association et al. as Amici Curiae Supporting Plaintiff-Appellees, *Perry v. Schwarzenegger*, 591 F.3d 1126 (9th Cir. Dec. 10, 2009) (No. 10-16696), Civil Case No. 09-CV-2292, http://www.apa.org/about/offices/ogc/amicus/perry.pdf; and *Hollingsworth v. Perry*, No. 12-144 (9th Cir. June 26, 2013), https://www.supremecourt.gov/opinions/12pdf/12-144_8oko.pdf.

3. Maya's partner prefers to use the pronouns *he, his,* and *him* or *they* and *them.*

4. The case (State of Kansas Department for Children and Families v. W.M.) involves an Indiana lesbian married couple that wanted both mothers' names on their child's birth certificate. According to reports, Judge Diane Sykes asserted biological parentage is primary: "If the

state defines parenthood by virtue of biology, no argument under the Equal Protection Clause or the substantive due process clause can overcome that" (https://www.usatoday.com/story /news/politics/2017/05/23/same-sex-birth-parents/339148001/). The State of Indiana is appealing a ruling by a district judge who sided with the same-sex couple and ordered the state to recognize both women as parents on birth certificates of children who are conceived through a sperm donor. For more information about the case, see (https://ecf.insd.uscourts .gov/cgi-bin/show_public_doc?12015cv0220-116).

5. Marisa N. Pavan et al. v. Nathaniel Smith, 582 U.S. (June 26, 2017) (per curiam), https:// www.supremecourt.gov/opinions/16pdf/16-992_868c.pdf.

6. Turner v. Oakley, No. 1 CA-SA 17-0028 (Ariz. Ct. App. filed June 22, 2017), http://www .azcourts.gov/Portals/0/OpinionFiles/Div1/2017/1%20CA-SA%2017-0028.pdf.

7. Loving v. Virginia, 388 U.S. 1 (1967), https://casetext.com/case/loving-v-commonwealth -of-virginia.

8. Thomas Beatie underwent partial sexual reassignment surgery, known as "top surgery," as an adult in 2002 but kept his ovaries and uterus. In 2003 in Hawaii, he and his wife married and he was legally recognized as a man. Beatie gave birth to three children between 2008 and 2010. In February 2012, he went through "bottom surgery" to finish his transition to male. Beatie then filed for legal separation from his wife in March 2012, and she filed for divorce. Arizona Superior Court judge Douglas Gerlach ruled that he had a lack of jurisdiction and could not grant the divorce because Arizona did not have to comply with out-of-state birth or marriage certificates and did not see hormone treatment and sexual reassignment surgery as proving Beatie was legally male. Since same-sex marriages were not permitted at the time, in the judge's opinion the two were not legally married. In 2014, Beatie appealed and was awarded divorce and custody of his children. See Emery (2012).

9. See Jessi Hempel's (2016) article about his experience.

10. See Liam Stack's (2017) *New York Times* article on this.

CHAPTER 10   CONCLUSION

1. Obergefell v. Hodges, 576 U.S. (2015).

2. Marisa N. Pavan et al. v. Nathaniel Smith, 582 U.S. (June 26, 2017).

3. For more information about my research on egg donors, see http://eggdonorresearch .org. I am also producing and directing a documentary film on egg donation. See http:// theperfectdonor.com for more information.

4. Michal Nahman and I are currently working on a forthcoming special edition on these issues, titled: *Beyond Bioavailable Bodies: Reproductive Work and Cross-Border Family Making,* for *Body and Society.*

REFERENCES

Abu-Lughod, Lila. 1993. *Writing Women's Worlds: Bedouin Stories*. Berkeley: University of California Press.

Agigian, Amy. 2004. *Baby Steps: How Lesbian Alternative Insemination Is Changing the World*. Middletown, CT: Wesleyan University Press.

Aizley, Harlyn. 2003. *Buying Dad: One Woman's Search for the Perfect Sperm Donor*. Los Angeles: Alyson Books.

Allan, Sonia. 2016. *Donor Conception and the Search for Information: From Secrecy to Openness*. London: Routledge.

Allison, Anne. 1994. *Nightwork: Sexuality, Pleasure, and Corporate Masculinity in a Tokyo Hostess Bar*. Chicago: University of Chicago Press.

Almeling, Rene. 2011. *Sex Cells: The Medical Market for Eggs and Sperm*. Berkeley: University of California Press.

———. 2017. "The Business of Egg and Sperm Donation." In *Contexts*, 6 (4): 68–70.

Alter, Joseph. 1997. "Seminal Truth: A Modern Science of Male Celibacy in Northern India." *Medical Anthropology Quarterly* 11 (3): 275–298.

Appadurai, Arjun. 1986. *The Social Life of Things: Commodities in Cultural Perspective*. Cambridge: Cambridge University Press.

Aprilia. n.d. "Fantasy (Sperm Donation)." AdForum, accessed June 20, 2018. https://www .adforum.com/creative-work/ad/player/1588/fantasy-sperm-donation/aprilia.

Arditti, Rita, Renate Duelli Klein, and Shelley Minden, eds. 1984. *Test-Tube Women: What Future for Motherhood?* London: Pandora.

Baylis, Francis. 2013. "The Ethics of Creating Children with Three Genetic Parents." *Reproductive Biomedicine Online* 26 (6): 531–534.

Becker, Gay. 1990. *Healing the Infertile Family*. New York: Bantam.

———. 1994. "Metaphors in Disrupted Lives: Infertility and Cultural Constructions of Continuity." *Medical Anthropology Quarterly* 8 (4): 383–410.

———. 1999. *Disrupted Lives: How People Create Meaning in a Chaotic World*. Berkeley: University of California Press.

———. 2000. *The Elusive Embryo*. Berkeley: University of California Press.

Beeson, Diane, and Abby Lippman. 2006. "Egg Harvesting for Stem Cell Research: Medical Risks and Ethical Problems." In *Reproductive Biomedicine Online* 13 (4): 573–579.

Beeson, Diane, P. K. Jennings, and Wendy Kramer. 2011. "Offspring Searching for Their Sperm Donors: How Family Type Shapes the Process." *Human Reproduction* 26 (9): 2415–2424.

Benintendi, Allyn. 2017. "Freezing the Future: Oocyte Cryopreservation in Northern California." Senior honors' thesis, University of California, Berkeley.

Benjamin, Ruha. 2013. *People's Science: Bodies and Rights on the Stem Cell Frontier*. Stanford, CA: Stanford University Press.

Berggren, C. 1997. "Sweden." In *Lesbian Motherhood in Europe*, edited by Kate Griffin and Lisa Mulholland. London: Cassell.

Biblarz, Timothy J., and Judith Stacey. 2010. "How Does the Gender of Parents Matter?" *Journal of Marriage and the Family* 72 (1): 3–22.

Bordo, Susan. 1993. *Unbearable Weight: Feminism, Western Culture and the Body*. Berkeley: University of California Press.

Bourdieu, Pierre. 1977. *Outline of a Theory of Practice*. Cambridge: Cambridge University Press.

Brandes, Stanley. 1987. *Forty: The Age and the Symbol*. Knoxville: University of Tennessee Press.

Brewer, Paul. 2003. "The Shifting Foundations of Public Opinion about Gay Rights." *Journal of Politics* 65 (4): 1208–1220.

Bull, Chris. 1993. "A Mother's Nightmare." *The Advocate*, 640:24–27.

Burgess, Ernest, and Harvey Locke. 1945. *The Family: From Institution to Companionship*. New York: American Book.

Cahn, Naomi, and June Carbone. 2003. "Which Ties Bind? Redefining the Parent-Child Relationship in the Age of Genetic Certainty." *William and Mary Bill of Rights Journal* 11 (3): 1011–1070.

Cannell, Fenella. 1990. "Concepts of Parenthood: The Warnock Report, the Gillick Debate and Modern Myths." *American Ethnologist* 17:667–686.

Cenziper, Debbie, and Jim Obergefell. 2016. *Love Wins: The Lovers and Lawyers Who Fought the Landmark Case for Marriage Equality*. New York: William Morrow.

Chan, Raymond W., Barbara Raboy, and Charlotte J. Patterson. 1998. "Psychosocial Adjustment among Children Conceived via Donor Insemination by Lesbian and Heterosexual Mothers." *Child Development* 69 (2): 443–457.

Cherlin, Andrew. 2004. "The Deinstitutionalization of Marriage." *Journal of Marriage and Family* 66:848–861.

Cohen, Lawrence. 1999. "The History of Semen: Notes on a Culture-Bound Syndrome." In *Medicine and the History of the Body*, edited by Yatsuo Otsuka, Shizu Sahai, and Shigehisa Kuriyama, 113–138. Tokyo: Ishiyaku Euro-American.

———. 2004. "Operability, Bioavailability and Exception." In *Global Assemblages: Technology, Politics, and Ethics as Anthropological Problems*, edited by Aihwa Ong and Stephen J. Collier, 79–90. Malden, MA: Blackwell.

Collins, Patricia Hill. 2015. "Intersectionality's Definitional Dilemmas." *Annual Review of Sociology* 41:1–20.

Collins, Patricia Hill, and Sirma Bilge. 2016. *Intersectionality*. Key Concepts. Cambridge: Polity.

Coontz, Stephanie. 2005. *Marriage, a History: How Love Conquered Marriage*. New York: Viking Penguin.

Cooper, Melinda, and Catherine Waldby. 2014. *Clinical Labor: Tissue Donors and Research Subjects in the Global Bioeconomy*. Durham, NC: Duke University Press.

Corea, Gena. 1985. *The Mother Machine: Reproductive Technologies from Artificial Insemination to Artificial Wombs*. New York: Harper and Row.

Corea, Gena, and Renate Duelli Klein. 1985. *Man-Made Women: How New Reproductive Technologies Affect Women*. London: Hutchinson.

Crenshaw, Kimberle. 1989. "Demarginalizing the Intersections of Race and Sex: A Black Feminist Critique of Antidiscrimination Doctrine, Feminist Theory and Anti-Racist Policies." *University of Chicago Legal Forum* 1989 (1): 139–167.

Cromer, Risa. 2017. "Waiting: The Redemption of Frozen Embryos through Embryo Adoption and Stem Cell Research in the United States." In *Anthropology of the Fetus: Biology, Culture, and Society*, edited by Sallie Han, Tracy Bestinger, and Amy Scott, 171–199. New York: Berghahn Books.

Culhane, John. 2015. "Sperm Donors Are Winning Visitation Rights." *Slate*, February 20, 2015. http://www.slate.com/articles/news_and_politics/jurisprudence/2015/02/sperm_donor _parental_rights_new_jersey_lesbian_couple_is_losing_visitation.html.

Daniels, Ken. 2001. "Sharing Information with Donor Insemination Offspring: A Child-Conception versus a Family-Building Approach." *Human Reproduction* 16 (9): 1792–1796.

Darnovsky, Marcy. 2013. "A Slippery Slope to Human Germline Modification." *Nature* 499 (7457): 127.

Davis-Floyd, Robbie. 2004. *Birth as an American Right of Passage*. Berkeley: University of California Press.

Davis-Floyd, Robbie, and Joseph Dumit, eds. 1998. *Cyborg Babies: From Techno-Sex to Techno-Tots*. New York: Routledge.

Dawkins, Richard. 1976. *The Selfish Gene*. Oxford: Oxford University Press.

De Zordo, Silvia, and Milena Marchesi, eds. 2015. *Reproduction and Biopolitics: Ethnographies of Governance, "Irrationality" and Resistance*. New York: Routledge.

Dice, Harry. 1994. "Speaking with Robert Klark Graham about the Genius Sperm Bank 3" (interview). https://www.youtube.com/watch?v=6Y79Kpy41YA.

Doan, Long, Annalise Loehr, and Lisa Miller. 2014. "Formal Rights and Informal Privileges for Same-Sex Couples." *American Sociological Review* 79 (6): 1172–1195.

Donovan, Catherine. 1997. "United Kingdom." In *Lesbian Motherhood in Europe*, edited by Kate Griffin and Lisa Mulholland, 217–224. London: Cassell.

Douglas, Mary. 1966. *Purity and Danger*. New York: Praeger.

———. 1968. *Pollution*. New York: Praeger.

———. 1970. *Natural Symbols*. New York: Pantheon.

Duster, Troy. 1990. *Backdoor to Eugenics*. New York: Routledge Chapman and Hall.

Edin, Kathryn, and Maria Kefalas. 2011. *Promises I Can Keep: Why Poor Women Put Motherhood before Marriage*. Berkeley: University of California Press.

Emery, Debbie. 2012. "'Pregnant Man' Thomas Beatie Opens Up about His Struggle to Have More Children." Radar, November 14, 2012. http://radaronline.com/exclusives/2012/11/pregnant-man-thomas-beatie-opens-struggle-more-children-anderson-cooper/.

Engels, Friedrich. [1884] 1972. *The Origin of the Family, Private Property, and the State*. Edited by Eleanor Leacock. New York: International.

Ethics Committee of the ASRM (American Society for Reproductive Medicine). 2004. "Informing Offspring of Their Conception by Gamete Donation." *Fertility and Sterility* 81 (3): 527–531.

———. 2006. "Access to Fertility Treatment by Gays, Lesbians, and Unmarried Persons." *Fertility and Sterility* 86 (5): 1333–1335.

———. 2013. "Access to Fertility Treatment by Gays, Lesbians, and Unmarried Persons: A Committee Opinion." *Fertility and Sterility* 100 (6): 1524–1527.

———. 2015. "Access to Fertility Services by Transgender Persons: An Ethics Opinion." *Fertility and Sterility* 104 (5): 1111–1115.

Evans-Pritchard, Edward E. (1937) 1976. *Witchcraft, Oracles, and Magic among the Azande*. Oxford: Oxford University Press.

Farmer, Paul. 1992. *AIDS and Accusation: Haiti and the Geography of Blame*. Berkeley: University of California Press.

Feminist Self-Insemination Group. 1980. *Self-Insemination*. London: Feminist Self-Insemination Group.

Finkler, Kaya. 2000. *Experiencing the New Genetics: Family and Kinship on the Medical Frontier*. Philadelphia: University of Pennsylvania Press.

Firestone, Shulamith. 1970. *The Dialectic of Sex: The Case for Feminist Revolution*. New York: William Morrow.

Flax, Jane. 1990. "Postmodernism and Gender Relations in Feminist Theory." In *Feminism/Postmodernism*, edited by Linda J. Nicholson, 39–62. New York: Routledge.

Fleming, A. T. 1980. "New Frontiers in Conception: Medical Breakthroughs and Moral Dilemmas." *New York Times Magazine*, July 20, 1980, 14–34, 42, 48.

Flower, Michael, and D. Heath. 1993. "Micro-anatomo Politics: Mapping the Human Genome Project." *Culture, Medicine, and Psychiatry* 17 (1): 27–42.

Forsythe, Diana. 1992. "Blaming the User in Medical Informatics: The Cultural Nature of Scientific Practice." In *Knowledge and Society: The Anthropology of Science and Technology*, edited by Linda L. Layne and David J. Hess, 9:95–111. Greenwich, CT: JAI.

Foucault, Michel. 1975. *Discipline and Punish: The Birth of the Prison*. New York: Vintage Books.

———.1980. *The History of Sexuality*. Vol. 1, *An Introduction*. New York: Random House, Vintage Books.

———.1988. *Technologies of the Self: A Seminar with Michel Foucault*, edited by Luther Hartman, Huck Gutman, and Patrick Hoffman. Amherst: University of Massachusetts Press.

———. 1990. *The History of Sexuality*. Vol. 2, *The Use of Pleasure*. New York: Vintage Books.

———. 2007. *Security, Territory, Population: Lectures at the College de France 1977–78*. Basingstoke, UK: Palgrave Macmillian.

Fox, Robin. 1967. *Kinship and Marriage*. Harmondsworth, UK: Pelican Books.

Frank, Katherine. 2002. *G-Strings and Sympathy: Strip Club Regulars and Male Desire*. Durham, NC: Duke University Press.

Franklin, Sarah. 1993. "Essentialism, Which Essentialism?" Some Implications of Genetic and Reproductive Technoscience. *Journal of Homosexuality* 24 (3–4): 27–40.

———. 1995. "Science as Culture, Cultures of Science." *Annual Review of Anthropology* 24:163–184.

———. 1997. *Embodied Progress: A Cultural Account of Assisted Reproduction*. New York: Routledge.

Franklin, Sarah, and Susan McKinnon. 2001. *Relative Values: Reconfiguring Kinship Studies*. Durham, NC: Duke University Press.

Franklin, Sarah, and Helena Ragone. 1998. *Reproducing Reproduction: Kinship, Power and Technological Innovation*. Philadelphia: University of Pennsylvania Press.

Freeman, Tabitha, Vasanti Jadva, Wendy Kramer, and Susan Golombok. 2009. "Gamete Donation: Parents' Experiences of Searching for their Child's Donor Siblings and Donor." In *Human Reproduction* 24 (3): 505–516.

Freeman, Tabitha, Sophie Zadeh, Vanessa Smith, and Susan Golombok. 2016. "Disclosure of Sperm Donation: A Comparison between Solo Mother and Two-Parent Families with Identifiable Donors. *Reproductive Biomedicine Online* 33 (5): 592–600.

Friese, Carrie, Gay Becker, and Robert Nachtigall. 2006. "Rethinking the Biological Clock: Eleventh Hour Moms, Miracle Moms, and Meanings of Age-Related Infertility." *Social Science and Medicine* 63 (6): 1550–1560.

Fulcher, Megan, Erin L. Sutfin, Raymond W. Chan, Joanna E. Scheib, and Charlotte J. Patterson. 2006. "Lesbian Mothers and Their Children: Findings from the Contemporary Families Study." In *Sexual Orientation and Mental Health: Examining Identity and Development in Lesbian, Gay, and Bisexual People*, edited by Allen M. Omoto and Howard S. Kurtzman, 281–299. Washington, DC: American Psychological Association.

Gailey, Christine Ward. 2010. *Blue-Ribbon Babies and Labors of Love: Race, Class and Gender in U.S. Adoption Practice*. Austin: University of Texas Press.

Gartrell, Nanette, and H. Boss. 2010. "US National Longitudinal Family Study: Psychological Adjustment of 17-Year-Old Adolescents." *Pediatrics* 126 (1): 28–36.

Gartrell, Nanette, Jean Hamilton, Amy Banks, Dee Mosbacher, Nancy Reed, Caroline H. Sparks, and Holly Bishop. 1996. "The National Lesbian Family Study: Interviews with Prospective Mothers." *American Journal of Orthopsychiatry* 66 (2): 272–281.

Gates, Gary J. 2014. LGB Families and Relationships: Analyses of the 2013 National Health Interview Survey. Los Angeles: Williams Institute, University of California, Los Angeles, School of Law. (https://williamsinstitute.law.ucla.edu/wp-content/uploads/lgb-families-nhis-sep-2014.pdf).

Geertz, Clifford. 1973. *The Interpretation of Cultures*. New York: Basic Books.

Ginsburg, Faye and Rayna Rapp, eds. 1995. *Conceiving the New World Order: The Global Politics of Reproduction*. Berkeley: University of California Press.

Goldberg, A. E., and Joanna Scheib. 2015. "Female-Partnered and Single Women's Contact Motivations and Experiences with Donor-Linked Families." *Human Reproduction* 30 (6): 1375–1385.

Golin, M. 1962. "Paternity by Proxy." *New Physician* 11:425–429.

Golombok, Susan. 2015. *Modern Families: Parents and Children in New Family Forms*. Cambridge: Cambridge University Press.

Graham, Robert K. 1970. *The Future of Man*. North Quincy, MA: Christopher.

Griffin, Kate, and Lisa Mulholland, eds. 1997. *Lesbian Motherhood in Europe*. London: Cassell.

Gupta, Jyotsna, and Annemiek Richters. 2008. "Embodied Subjects and Fragment Objects: Women's Bodies, Assisted Reproduction Technologies and the Rights to Self- Determination." *Journal of Bioethical Inquiry* 5 (4): 239–249.

Hanson, Allan. 1996. "Genetics and Personal Responsibility." Paper presented at the Ninety-Fifth Annual American Anthropological Association Meetings. San Francisco, CA, November.

Haraway, Donna. 1991. *Simians, Cyborgs and Women: The Reinvention of Nature*. New York: Routledge.

———. 1997. *Modest_Witness@Second_Millennium.FemaleMan©_Meets_ OncoMouse*. New York: Routledge.

Harrison, Laura. 2016. *Brown Bodies, White Babies: The Politics of Cross-Racial Surrogacy*. New York: New York University Press.

Hayden, Corinne. 1995. "Gender, Genetics and Generation: Reformulating Biology in Lesbian Kinship." *Cultural Anthropology* 10 (1): 41–63.

Hempel, Jessi. 2016. "My Brother's Pregnancy and the Making of a New American Family." *Time*, September 12, 2016. http://time.com/4475634/trans-man-pregnancy-evan/.

Herbst, Arthur L., Howard Ulfelder, and David C. Poskanzer. 1971. "Adenocarcinoma of the Vagina—Association of Maternal Stilbestrol Therapy with Tumor Appearance in Young Women." *New England Journal of Medicine* 284 (16): 878–881.

Herdt, Gilbert. 1981. *Guardians of the Flutes: Idioms of Masculinity*. New York: McGraw-Hill.

Hertz, Rosanna, Ana Maria Rivas, and Maria Isabel Rubio Jociles. 2016. "Single Mothers of Choice in Spain and the United States." In *The Wiley Blackwell Encyclopedia of Family Studies*, edited by Constance L. Shehan, 1812–1815. Hoboken, NJ: Wiley Blackwell.

Hochschild, Arlie. 1983. *The Managed Heart: Commercialization of Human Feeling*. Berkeley: University of California Press.

Holland, Maximilian. 2012. *Social Bonding and Nurture Kinship: Compatibility between Cultural and Biological Approaches*. Createspace Independent Publishing.

Hornstein, F. 1984. "Children by Donor Insemination: A New Choice for Lesbians." In *Test-Tube Women: What Future for Motherhood?*, edited by Rita Arditti, Renate Duelli Klein, and Shelley Minden, 373–381. London: Pandora.

Hubbard, Ruth. 1990. *The Politics of Women's Biology*. New Brunswick, NJ: Rutgers University Press.

Hubbard, Ruth, and Elijah Wald. 1993. *Exploding the Gene Myth*. Boston: Beacon.

Inhorn, Marcia. 1994. *Quest for Conception: Gender, Infertility, and Egyptian Medical Traditions*. Philadelphia: University of Pennsylvania Press.

———. 1995. *Infertility and Patriarchy: The Cultural Politics of Gender and Family Life in Egypt*. Philadelphia: University of Pennsylvania Press.

————, ed. 2007a. *Reproductive Disruptions: Gender, Technology, and Biopolitics in the New Millennium*. New York: Berghahn Books.

————.2007b. "Masturbation, Semen Collection and Men's IVF Experiences: Anxieties in the Muslim World." In "Islam, Health and the Body: Science and Religion in the Modern Muslim World, edited by Diane Tober and Debra Budiani. Special issue, *Body and Society* 13 (3): 37–53, London: Sage.

————. 2015. *Cosmopolitan Conceptions: IVF Sojourns in Global Dubai*. Durham, NC: Duke University Press.

Jiménez, Karleen Pendelton. 2011. *How to Get a Girl Pregnant*. Toronto: Zurita.

Kahn, Susan. 2000. *Reproducing Jews: A Cultural Account of Assisted Reproduction in Israel*. Durham, NC: Duke University Press.

Keller, Evelyn Fox. 1985. *Reflections on Gender and Science*. New Haven, CT: Yale University Press.

Kempadoo, Kamala. 1998. "Introduction: Globalizing Sex Workers' Rights." In *Global Sex Workers: Rights, Resistance, and Redefinition*, edited by Kamala Kempadoo and Jo Doezema, 1–29. New York: Routledge.

Kevles, Daniel. 1985. *In the Name of Eugenics: Genetics and the Uses of Human Heredity*. Berkeley: University of California Press.

Kimbrell, Andrew. 1993. *The Human Body Shop: The Engineering and Marketing of Life*. San Francisco: Harper.

Kimport, Katrina. 2014. *Queering Marriage*. New Brunswick, NJ: Rutgers University Press.

Klein, Renate Duelli. 1984. "Doing It Ourselves: Self-Insemination." In *Test-Tube Women: What Future for Motherhood?*, edited by Rita Arditti, Renate Duelli Klein, and Shelley Minden, 382–390. London: Pandora.

Konvalinka, Nancy. 2013. "Late-Forming Families, Life Course, and Generation in Spain Today." Unpublished conference paper.

Krause, Elizabeth, and Silvia de Zordo. 2012. "Introduction: Ethnography and Biopolitics: Tracing 'Rationalities' of Reproduction across the North–South Divide." In "Reproduction and Biopolitics," special issue, *Anthropology and Medicine* 19 (22): 137–151.

————. 2015. "Ethnography and Biopolitics: Tracing 'Rationalities' of Reproduction across the North-South Divide." Introduction to *Reproduction and Biopolitics: Ethnographies of Governance, "Irrationality" and Resistance*, edited by Silvia de Zordo and Milena Marchesi, 1–16. New York: Routledge.

Kritchevsky, B. 1981. "The Unmarried Woman's Right to Artificial Insemination: A Call for an Expanded Definition of Family." *Harvard Women's Law Journal* 4 (1): 1–42.

Kuhn, Thomas. 1963. *The Structure of Scientific Revolutions*. Chicago: University of Chicago Press.

Laquer, Thomas. 1990. *Making Sex*. Cambridge, MA: Harvard University Press.

Latour, Bruno, and Steven Woolgar. 1986. *Laboratory Life*. Princeton, NJ: Princeton University Press.

Layne, Linda. 1992. "Of Fetuses and Angels: Fragmentation and Integration in Narratives of Pregnancy Loss." In *Knowledge and Society: The Anthropology of Science and Technology*, edited by David Hess and Linda Layne, 29–58. Greenwich: JAI Press.

————.2003. *Motherhood Lost: A Feminist Account of Pregnancy Loss in America*. New York: Routledge.

Leacock, Eleanor Burke. 1972. Introduction to *The Origin of the Family, Private Property and the State: In the Light of the Researches of Lewis H. Morgan*, by Frederich Engels. New York: International Publishers Company.

Lehman-Haupt, Rachel. 2016. *In Her Own Sweet Time: Egg Freezing and the New Frontiers of Family*. San Francisco: Nothing but the Truth.

Lehr, Valerie. 1999. *Queer Family Values: Debunking the Myth of the Nuclear Family*. Philadelphia: Temple University Press.

Levi-Strauss, Claude. (1949) 1969. *The Elementary Structures of Kinship*. Revised edition, Boston: Beacon. Originally published in France as *Les Structures élémentaires de la Parenté*.

Lewin, Ellen. 1981. "Lesbianism and Motherhood: The Virgin Mary as Economic Woman" (with C. Browner). *American Ethnologist* 9 (1): 61–75.

———. 1993. *Lesbian Mothers: Accounts of Gender in American Culture*. Ithaca, NY: Cornell University Press.

———. 1998. "Queering Reproduction?" Paper presented at invited session, the Gendered Politics of Reproduction, C. H. Browner and C. Sargent, organizers, of the American Anthropological Association, Philadelphia.

———. 2009. *Gay Fatherhood: Narratives of Family and Citizenship in America*. Chicago: University of Chicago Press.

Lewin, Ellen, and T. A. Lyons. 1982. "Everything in Its Place: The Coexistence of Lesbianism and Motherhood." In *Homosexuality: Social Psychological and Biological Issues*, edited by W. Paul, J. D. Weinrich, J. C. Gonsiorek, and M. E. Hotvedt, 249–274. Beverly Hills: Sage.

Livingston, Gretchen. 2014. "Fewer Than Half of U.S. Kids Today Live in a 'Traditional' Family." Pew Research Center Report. http://www.pewresearch.org/fact-tank/2014/12/22/less-than-half-of-u-s-kids-today-live-in-a-traditional-family/.

Lock, Margaret, and Deborah Gordon. 1988. *Biomedicine Examined*. Dordrecht: Kluwer.

Lock, Margaret, and Shirley Lindenbaum. 1993. *Knowledge, Power, and Practice*. Berkeley: University of California Press.

Luna, Zakiya, and Kristin Luker. 2013. "Reproductive Justice." *Annual Reviews of Law and Social Science* 9:327–352.

Mac Dougall, Kristin; Gay Becker, Joanna Scheib, and Robert Nachtigall. 2007. "Strategies for Disclosure: How Parents Approach Telling Their Children That They Were Conceived with Donor Gametes." *Fertility and Sterility* 87 (3): 524–533.

Malinowski, Bronislaw. 1922. *Argonauts of the Western Pacific: An Account of Native Enterprise and Adventure in the Archipelagoes of Melanesian New Guinea*. London: Routledge and Kegan Paul.

Mamo, Laura. 2007. *Queering Reproduction: Achieving Pregnancy in the Age of Technoscience*. Durham, NC: Duke University Press.

Markens, Susan. 2007. *Surrogate Motherhood and the Politics of Reproduction*. Berkeley: University of California Press.

Marquardt, Elizabeth, Norval Glenn, and Karen Clark. 2010. *My Daddy's Name Is Donor*. New York: Institute for American Values.

Martin, Emily. 1987. *The Woman in the Body: A Cultural Analysis of Reproduction*. Boston: Beacon.

———. 1990. "The Ideology of Reproduction: The Reproduction of Ideology." In *Uncertain Terms: Negotiating Gender in American Culture*, edited by Faye Ginsburg and Anna Lowenhaupt Tsing, 300–314. Boston: Beacon.

———. 1991. "The Egg and the Sperm: How Science Has Constructed a Romance Based on Stereotypical Male-Female Roles." *Signs* 16:485–501.

———. 1994. *Flexible Bodies*. Boston: Beacon.

Marx, Karl. 1906. *Capitol*. New York: Modern Library.

Mattes, Jane. 1994. *Single Mothers by Choice: A Guidebook for Single Women Who Are Considering or Have Chosen Motherhood*. New York: Times Books.

Matthews, T. J., and Brady E. Hamilton. 2016. "Mean Age of Mothers Is on the Rise: United States, 2000–2014." NCHS Data Brief No. 232, January 2016. https://www.cdc.gov/nchs/data/databriefs/db232.htm.

Mauss, Marcel. 1954. *The Gift: Forms and Functions of Exchange in Archaic Societies*. London: Routledge.

Melhuus, Marit. 2012. *Problems of Conception: Issues of Law, Biotechnology, Individuals, and Kinship*. New York: Berghahn Books.

Merleau-Ponty, Maurice. 1944. *The Phenomenology of Perception*. London: Routledge.

Miller, Naomi. 1992. *Single Parents by Choice: A Growing Trend in Family Life*. New York: Insight Books.

Mills, Catherine. 2006. *Futures of Reproduction: Bioethics and Biopolitics*. New York: Springer.

Mitra, Sayani, and Sybille Lustenburger. Forthcoming. "Mobile Bodies, Desires, and Ideas: A Discussion on the Shifting Market of Commercial Surrogacy." In "Beyond Bioavailable Bodies: Reproductive Work and Cross-Border Family Making," edited by Diane Tober and Michal Nahman, special issue, *Body and Society*.

Modell, Judith. 1994. *Kinship with Strangers: Adoption and Interpretations of Kinship in American Culture*. Berkeley: University of California Press.

Mohr, Sebastian. 2014. "Beyond Motivation: On What It Means to Be a Sperm Donor in Denmark." *Anthropology and Medicine* 21 (2): 162–173.

———. 2016. "Containing Sperm—Managing Legitimacy: Lust, Disgust, and Hybridity at Danish Sperm Banks." *Journal of Contemporary Ethnography* 45 (3): 319–342.

Moore, Lisa Jean. 2007. *Sperm Counts: Overcome by Man's Most Precious Fluid*. New York: New York University Press.

Moore, Mignon. 2011. *Invisible Families: Gay Identities, Relationships, and Motherhood among Black Women*. Berkeley: University of California Press.

Morgan, Lewis Henry. 1871. *Systems of Consanguinity and Affinity of the Human Family*. Washington, DC: Smithsonian.

Morsy, Soheir. 1990. "Biotechnology and the International Politics of Population Control: Long-Term Contraception in Egypt." In *Signs*.

Mosher, William, and William Pratt. 1982. *Fecundity, Infertility, and Reproductive Health in the United States*. Washington, DC: U.S. Department of Health and Human Services, National Center for Health Statistics.

Muller, Hermann. 1950. Our Load of Mutations." *American Journal of Human Genetics* 2:111–176.

———.1959. "The Guidance of Human Evolution." *Perspectives in Biology and Medicine* 3:1–43.

———.1962. *Studies in Genetics: Selected Papers of H. J. Muller*. Bloomington: Indiana University Press.

Nachtigall, Robert, Gay Becker, and Mark Wozny. 1992. "The Effects of Gender-Specific Diagnosis in Men's and Women's Response to Infertility." *Fertility and Sterility* 57 (1): 113–121.

Nachtigall, Robert, Jeanne Tschann, Selize Quiroga, Linda Pitcher, and Gay Becker. 1997. "Stigma, Disclosure and Family Functioning among Parents of Children Conceived through Donor Insemination." *Fertility and Sterility* 68 (1): 83–89.

Nader, Laura. 1972. "Up the Anthropologist: Perspectives Gained from Studying Up." In *Reinventing Anthropology*, edited by Dell Hymes, 284–311. Ann Arbor: University of Michigan Press.

———. 1996. *Naked Science: Boundaries, Power, and Knowledge*. London: Routledge.

Nahman, Michal. 2016. "Romanian IVF: A Brief History through the Lens of Labour, Migration, and Global Egg Donation Markets." *Reproductive Biomedicine and Society* 2:79–87.

Noble, David F. 1977. *America by Design: Science, Technology, and the Rise of Corporate Capitalism*. Oxford: Oxford University Press.

Obasogie, Osagie, and Marcy Darnovsky. 2018. *Beyond Bioethics: Toward a New Biopolitics*. Berkeley: University of California Press.

Ong, Aihwa, and Stephen J. Collier. 2004. *Global Assemblages: Technology, Politics, and Ethics as Anthropological Problems*. Malden, MA: Blackwell.

Pasch, Lauri, Jean Benward, Joanna Scheib, and Julia Wooward. 2017. "Donor-Conceived Children: The View Ahead." *Human Reproduction* 32 (7): 1234.

Pelka, Suzanne. 2009. "Sharing Motherhood: Maternal Jealousy and Lesbian Co-mothers." *Journal of Homosexuality* 56 (2): 195–217.

Perry, Samuel, and Andrew Whitehead. 2016. "Religion and Public Opinion toward Same-Sex Relations, Marriage, and Adoption: Does the Type of Practice Matter?" *Journal for the Scientific Study of Religion* 55 (3): 637–651.

Persaud, Sherina, Tabitha Freeman, Vasanti Jadva, Jenna Slutsky, Wendy Kramer, Miriam Steele, Howard Steele, and Susan Golombok. 2017. "Adolescents Conceived through Donor Insemination in Mother-Headed Families: A Qualitative Study of Motivations and Experiences of Contacting and Meeting Same-Donor Offspring." *Children and Society* 31 (1): 13–22.

Pilpel, Harriet F. 1985. "New Methods of Conception and Their Legal Status." *New York Law School Human Rights Annual* 3 (Fall): 1–33.

Plotz, David. 2005. *The Genius Factory: The Curious History of the Nobel Prize Sperm Bank*. New York: Random House.

Polakow, Valerie. 1993. *Lives on the Edge: Single Mothers and Their Children in the Other America*. Chicago: University of Chicago Press.

Rabinow, Paul. 1992. "Artificiality and Enlightenment: From Sociobiology to Biosociality." In *Zone*, vol. 6, *Incorporations*, edited by Jonathan Crary and Sanford Kwinter, 234–252. New York: Zone.

———. 1993. "Galton's Regret and DNA Typing." *Culture, Medicine and Psychiatry* 17 (1): 59–65.

Radcliffe-Brown, A. R. 1922. *The Andaman Islanders*. Cambridge: Cambridge University Press.

Ragone, Helena. 1994. *Surrogate Motherhood: Conceptions in the Heart*. Boulder: Westview Press.

Rapp, Rayna. 1988. "Chromosomes and Communication: The Discourse of Genetic Counseling." *Medical Anthropology Quarterly* 2 (2): 143–157.

———. 1999. *Testing Women, Testing the Fetus: The Social Impact of Amniocentesis in America*. New York: Routledge.

Reich, Jennifer. 2005. *Fixing Families: Parents, Power, and the Child Welfare System*. New York: Routledge.

"Reproductive Technology and the Procreation Rights of the Unmarried." 1985. Notes, *Harvard Law Review* 98 (3): 669–685.

Rich, Adrienne. 1980. "Compulsory Heterosexuality and Lesbian Existence." *Signs* 5 (4): 631–660.

———. 1986. *Of Woman Born*. New York: W. W. Norton.

Richards, Sarah Elizabeth. 2013. *Motherhood Rescheduled: The New Frontier of Egg Freezing and the Women Who Tried It*. New York: Simon and Schuster.

Roberts, Dorothy. 1998. *Killing the Black Body: Race, Reproduction and the Meaning of Liberty*. New York: Vintage.

Roberts, Elizabeth. 1998. "Examining Surrogacy Discourses between Feminine Power and Exploitation." In *Small Wars: The Cultural Politics of Childhood*, edited by Nancy Scheper-Hughes and Carolyn Sargent, 93–109. Berkeley: University of California Press.

Rohleder, Hermann. 1994. *Test Tube Babies: A History of the Artificial Impregnation of Human Beings*. New York: Panurge.

Ross, Loretta, and Rickie Solinger. 2017. *Reproductive Justice: A New Vision for the 21st Century*. Berkeley: University of California Press.

Rubin, Gayle. 1975. "Traffic in Women: Notes on the 'Political Economy' of Sex." In *Toward an Anthropology of Women*, edited by Rayna Rapp Reiter, 157–210. New York: Monthly Review.

————. 1984. "Thinking Sex." In *Pleasure and Danger: Exploring Female Sexuality*, edited by Carole S. Vance, 143–178. Boston: Routledge and Kegan Paul.

Sacks, Karen. 1975. "Engels Revisited: Women, the Organization of Production and Private Property." In *Woman, Culture, and Society*, edited by Michell Zimbalist Rosaldo and Louise Lamphere, 207–222. Stanford, CA: Stanford University Press.

Said, Edward. 1978. *Orientalism*. New York: Vintage Books.

Sandelowski, Margarete. 1993. *With Child in Mind: Studies of the Personal Encounter with Infertility*. Philadelphia: University of Pennsylvania Press.

Sapir, E. 1961. *Culture, Language and Personality: Selected Essays*. Edited by David G. Mandelbaum. Berkeley: University of California Press.

Sargent, Carolyn, and Grace Bascope. 1996. "Ways of Knowing about Birth in Three Cultures." *Medical Anthropology Quarterly* 10 (2): 213–236.

Scheib, Joanna E., and Paul D. Hastings. 2012. "Donor-Conceived Children Raised by Lesbian Couples: Socialization and Development in a New Form of Planned Family." In *Families: Beyond the Nuclear Ideal*, edited by Daniela Cutas and Sarah Chan, 64–83. London: Bloomsbury Academic.

Scheib, Joanna E., M. Riordan, and S. Rubin. 2005. "Adolescents with Open-Identity Sperm Donors: Reports from 12–17 Year Olds." *Human Reproduction* 20 (1): 239–252.

Scheib, Joanna E., Alice Ruby, and Jean Benward. 2017. "Who Requests Their Sperm Donor's Identity? The First 10 Years of Information Releases to Adults with Open-Identity Donors." *Fertility and Sterility* 107 (2): 483–493.

Schellan, A. 1957. *Artificial Insemination in the Human*. Amsterdam: Elsevier.

Scheper-Hughes, Nancy. 1985. "Science and Gender: A Critique of Biology and Its Theories on Women." *Feminist Issues*, Spring, 80–92.

————. 1992. *Death without Weeping*. Berkeley: University of California Press.

————. 2000. "Global Traffic in Organs. *Current Anthropology* 41 (2): 191–224.

————. 2002. "Bodies for Sale—Whole or in Parts." In Commodifying Bodies, edited by Nancy Scheper-Hughes and Loic Wacquant. London: Sage.

————. 2007. The Tyranny of the Gift: Sacrificial Violence in Living Donor Transplants. *American Journal of Transplantation* 7 (3): 507–511.

Scheper-Hughes, Nancy, and Margaret Lock. 1987. "The Mindful Body: A Prolegomenon to Future Work in Medical Anthropology." *Medical Anthropology Quarterly* 18 (1): 6–41.

Scherman, Rhoda, Gabriela Misca, Karen Rotabi, and Peter Selman. 2016. "Global Commercial Surrogacy and International Adoption: Parallels and Differences." *Adoption and Fostering* 40 (1): 20–35.

Schneider, David. 1968. *American Kinship: A Cultural Account*. Englewood Cliffs, NJ: Prentice-Hall.

————. 1984. *A Critique of the Study of Kinship*. Ann Arbor: University of Michigan Press.

Schneider, Jennifer, Jennifer Lahl, and Wendy Kramer. (2017). "Long-term Breast Cancer Risk Following Ovarian Stimulation in Young Egg Donors: A Call for Follow-up, Research, and Informed Consent." *Reproductive Biomedicine Online* 34 (5): 480–485.

Serwer, Adam. 2012. "Ann Romney and the Subversive Conservatism of ABS's 'Modern Family.'" *Mother Jones*, August 29, 2012. http://www.motherjones.com/politics/2012/08/ann-romney -and-subversive-conservatism-abcs-modern-family/.

Shanley, Mary Lyndon, and Adrienne Asch. 2009. "Involuntary Childlessness, Reproductive Technology, and Social Justice: The Medical Mask on Social Illness." *Signs* 34 (4): 851–874.

Shapiro, E. Donald, and Lisa Schultz. 1990. "Single-Sex Families: The Impact of Birth Innovations upon Traditional Family Notions." *Journal of Family Law* 24 (2): 271–281.

Sharp, Lesley. 1995. "Organ Donation as a Transformative Experience." *Medical Anthropology Quarterly* 9 (3): 357–389.

Shore, Chris. 1992. "From Virgin Births to Sterile Debates: Anthropology and the New Reproductive Technologies." *Current Anthropology* 33:295–314.

Silliman, Jael, Marlene Gerber Fried, Loretta Ross, and Elena Gutiérrez. 2004. *Undivided Rights: Women of Color Organize for Reproductive Justice.* Cambridge, MA: South End Press.

Snowden, Robert, Geoffrey Duncan Mitchell, and E. M. Snowden. 1983. *Artificial Reproduction: A Social Investigation.* London: Allen and Unwin.

Solinger, Rickie. 2013. *Reproductive Politics: What Everyone Needs to Know.* Oxford: Oxford University Press.

Speier, Amy. 2016. *Fertility Holidays: IVF Tourism and the Reproduction of Whiteness.* New York: New York University Press.

Sperm Bank of California, The. 1991. Annual Report.

Stacey, Judith. 1990. *Brave New Families: Stories of Domestic Upheaval in Late-Twentieth-Century America.* Berkeley: University of California Press.

Stack, Carol. 1974. *All Our Kin.* New York: Harper and Row.

Stack, Liam. 2017. "European Court Strikes Down Required Sterilization for Transgender People." *New York Times,* April 12, 2017. https://www.nytimes.com/2017/04/12/world/europe/european-court-strikes-down-required-sterilization-for-transgender-people.html.

Stanworth, Michelle, ed. 1987. *Reproductive Technologies: Gender, Motherhood and Medicine.* Minneapolis: University of Minnesota Press.

Stern, S. 1980. "Lesbian Insemination." *Co-evolution Quarterly,* Summer, 108–117.

Stotzer, Rebecca L., Jody L. Herman, and Amira Hasenbush. 2014. *Transgender: A Review of Existing Research.* Los Angeles: Williams Institute, University of California, Los Angeles, School of Law. http://williamsinstitute.law.ucla.edu/wp-content/uploads/transgender-parenting-oct-2014.pdf.

Strathern, Marilyn. 1992a. *After Nature: English Kinship in the Late Twentieth Century.* Cambridge: Cambridge University Press.

———. 1992b. *Reproducing the Future: Anthropology, Kinship and the New Reproductive Technologies.* New York: Routledge.

Sullivan, Maureen, 2004. *The Family of Woman.* Berkeley: University of California Press.

Thompson, Charis. 2005. *Making Parents: The Ontological Choreography of Reproductive Technologies.* Cambridge, MA: MIT Press.

Thorne, Barrie, and Marilyn Yalom. 1982. *Rethinking the Family: Some Feminist Questions.* Boston: Northeastern University Press.

Titmuss, Richard. (1970) 1997. *The Gift Relationship: From Human Blood to Social Policy.* Edited by Ann Oakley and John Ashton. Expanded ed. New York: New Press.

Tober, Diane. 2002. "Semen as Gift, Semen as Goods: Reproductive Workers and the Market in Altruism." In *Commodifying Bodies,* edited by Nancy Scheper-Hughes and Loïc Wacquant, 137–160. London: Sage.

———. 2018. "Feminist Paradoxes." In "Once and Future Feminist," edited by Deborah Chasman and Joshua Cohen, 57–60. *Boston Review.*

Tober, Diane, and Vincenzo Pavone. 2018. "Bioeconomies of Egg Provision in the United States and Spain: Comparing Medical Markets and Implications for Donor Care." Original paper to be published in *Spanish Monográfico Ras,* edited by Ana María Rivas and Consuelo Álvarez, 2018, 27 (2).

Towghi, F. 2013. "The Biopolitics of Reproductive Technologies beyond the Clinic: Localizing HPV Vaccines in India." *Medical Anthropology* 32 (4): 325–342.

Tremayne, Soraya, and Marcia Inhorn. 2012. *Islam and Assisted Reproductive Technologies.* New York: Berghahn Books.

Twine, France Winddance. 2011. *Outsourcing the Womb: Race, Class, and Gestational Surrogacy in a Global Market.* New York: Routledge.

U.S. Congress, Office of Technology Assessment. 1988. *Infertility: Medical and Social Choices.* OTA-BA-358. Washington, DC: U.S. Government Printing Office.

Van Steirteghem, Andre. 2012. "Celebrating ICSI's Twentieth Anniversary and the Birth of More Than 2.5 Million Children—The 'How, Why, When and Where.'" *Human Reproduction* 27 (1): 1–2.

Varley, Emma. 2012. "Islamic Logics, Reproductive Rationalities: Family Planning in Northern Pakistan." *Anthropology and Medicine* 19 (2): 189–206.

Wajcman, Judy. 1991. *Feminism Confronts Technology.* University Park: Pennsylvania State University Press.

Waldby, Catherine, and Melinda Cooper. 2008. "The Biopolitics of Reproduction: Post-Fordist Biotechnology and Women's Clinical Labour." *Australian Feminist Studies* 23 (55): 57–73.

Wang, Stephanie. 2017. "Judge to Indiana Same-Sex Couples: 'You Can't Overcome Biology.'" *Indianapolis Star,* May 23, 2017. http://www.indystar.com/story/news/politics/2017/05/23/judge-indiana-same-sex-couples-you-cant-overcome-biology/338215001/.

Weber, Max. (1910) 1971. Max Weber on Race and Society. Translated. *Social Research* 38:30–41.

———. (1922) 1968. *Economy and Society.* Translated and edited by G. Roth and C. Wittich. New York: Bedminster.

Weston, Kath. (1991) 1997. *Families We Choose: Lesbian, Gays, Kinship.* Rev. ed. New York: Columbia University Press.

———. 1995. "Forever Is a Long Time: Romancing the Real in Gay Kinship Terminology." In *Naturalizing Power: Essays in Feminist Cultural Analysis,* edited by Sylvia Yanagisako and Carol DeLaney, 87–110. New York: Routledge.

Whitehead, Andrew, and Samuel Perry. 2015. "A More Perfect Union? Christian Nationalism and Support for Same-Sex Unions." *Sociological Perspectives* 58 (3): 422–440.

———. 2016. "Religion and Support for Adoption by Same-Sex Couples: The Relative Effects of Religious Tradition, Practices, and Beliefs." *Journal of Family Issues* 37 (6): 789–813.

Whorf, Benjamin Lee. 1956. *Language, Thought and Reality. Selected Writings.* Edited by John B. Carroll. Cambridge, MA: MIT Press.

Wolf, Deborah C. 1982. "Lesbian Childbirth and Artificial Insemination: A Wave of the Future." In *Anthropology of Human Birth,* edited by Margarita A. Kay, 321–339. Philadelphia: F. A. Davis.

Yanagisako, Sylvia, and Carol DeLaney, eds. 1995. *Naturalizing Power: Essays in Feminist Cultural Analysis,* 1–24. New York: Routledge.

Young, Katharine. 1997. *Presence in the Flesh: The Body in Medicine.* Cambridge, MA: Harvard University Press.

Zelizer, Viviana A. 1994. *Pricing the Priceless Child.* Princeton, NJ: Princeton University Press.

INDEX

abstinence, sperm donors and, 69, 94. *See also* sexuality

Abu-Lughod, Lila, 8

access to care: biopolitics and, 188–190; health insurance and, 182–184; lesbian baby boom and, 33–35; for single men and gay couples, 186–187; for single women and lesbian couples, 17–19, 27–29, 106–111, 127, 132, 158–160, 168, 177

adoption: "alternative" family and, 155; child custody and, 13; embryos and, 177; and international, 171, 182, 186, 191; open, 152; as pathway to parenthood, 106, 115, 170; reproductive politics and, 4; same-sex couples and, 169; second parent, 37, 47–50, 122, 157, 162; transracial, 92

advertising: egg v. sperm donor, 103; money, altruism, and, 91, 94; sexuality and, 51; sperm bank donor recruitment and, 51, 66, 88; women to find donors online, 35, 37

agency, 13, 18, 187–189

AIDS: donor screening and, 61–63; donor sexuality and, 69; fresh semen and, 60, 97; "geography of blame" and, 52–53; known donors and, 35–37, 150; LGBTQ family formation and, 134, 146, 175; rise of sperm banks and, 19, 186; risk and, 52; sperm bank regulations and, 55–57; sperm-washing and, 176, 187. *See also* HIV/AIDS

Almeling, Rene, 9, 89

altruism: commodification of, 86–89, 97–101, 102–104; donor choice and, 12, 151; donor motivations and, 60, 68, 94–99, 102; framing of, 69; genetic continuation and, 101; genetic inheritance and, 21–24; social/moral value of, 21, 104; sperm v. egg donors, gender and, 88–91

American Society for Reproductive Medicine (ASRM), ethics and LGBTQ access to treatment, 110–111, 113, 158, 179, 183

anonymity: appointment scheduling and, 26; child identity and, 152–155; donor, 2, 5, 7; and donor selection, 39–40, 149; "gift" and, 97; known donors and, 71–73, 94, 152; mandatory anonymity in Spain, 16; open-identity donors and, 96–97, 180; perceptions of fatherhood and, 50; secrecy and, 179; sperm bank approaches to, 29, 35

Appadurai, Arjun, 91–92

assisted reproduction and assisted reproductive technologies (ARTs): anthropological studies of, 9, 156; biopolitics and, 185–188; HIV/AIDS, homophobia and, 36; masculinity and, 54; marriage equality and, 163; new kin terminologies and, 181; personhood, kinship and, 14; single mother and LGBTQ access to, 3, 17, 20, 158, 160–166, 169–173

Beatie, Thomas, 173

Becker, Gay, 7, 8, 32, 105, 126

biogenetic, 130

biological versus social kinship. *See* kinship

biopolitechs, 185–188

biopolitics, 3–9, 160, 188

biopower, 3, 133, 188

biosociality, 13, 75

body: anthropology of, 10–13; commodification of, 190; female body, 33; infertility, failure and, 105–108, 116–118, 119–128; insemination and heightened awareness of, 30–31, 85; phenomenology of exchange and, 93; reproductive work and, 101–103; as site of labor, 88; sperm donation and sexual body, 63–66; transgender identity, non-binary gender and, 172–179

body commodification, 78, 88, 97, 101–103, 190. *See also* body: commodification of

Bourdieu, Pierre, 91

Center for Disease Control (CDC), 55–60

child custody, 3, 13, 37; fear of losing, 140, 149; known donors and, 15, 140, 146; known donors fighting for, 160–162; LGBTQ people and, 133, 157, 175–176, 185, 201n8; non-biological mom and custody, 46–48

cisgender, 9. *See also* gender

Cohen, Lawrence, 53, 54, 188, 190

ABOUT THE AUTHOR

DIANE TOBER is an assistant adjunct professor at the University of California, San Francisco, Institute for Health and Aging. She is a cultural and medical anthropologist with a focus on gender and sexuality, the commodification of the body, science and technology studies, bioethics, and social and reproductive justice. She has conducted ethnographic fieldwork in Iran, Spain, and the United States. Her research has been supported by the National Science Foundation, the Social Science Research Council, and the University of California, San Francisco, among others. With funding from the National Science Foundation, her current research explores the effects of culture on human biomarkets. For this work she is focusing on egg donation in the United States and Spain—two countries with vastly different regulatory approaches to third-party reproduction. In addition to her research, she is currently working on several documentary film projects on the international human egg market.

Printed and bound by CPI Group (UK) Ltd, Croydon, CR0 4YY

16/04/2025

14658332-0002

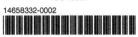